Fetish Sex

Fetish Sex

An Erotic Guide for Couples

by Violet Blue

Stories by Thomas Roche

Daedalus Publishing

PUBLISHED IN THE UNITED STATES BY DAEDALUS PUBLISHING
2807 W. SUNSET BLVD., LOS ANGELES, CA 90026
213-484-3882
INFO@DAEDALUSPUBLISHING.COM

PRINTED IN THE UNITED STATES.
EROTIC STORIES: THOMAS ROCHE
COVER DESIGN: STEVE DIET GOEDDE
COVER PHOTOGRAPH: STEVE DIET GOEDDE
TEXT DESIGN: ANGELA FAITH BROWN
FIRST EDITION.
10 9 8 7 6 5 4 3 2 1

Contents

trampling, and being crushed • Balloons and looners • Human mannequins and robots • Midgets • Tickling • Sleeping • Carrying, or "lift and carry" • Necrophilia

Introduction
Confessions of a Fetishist

About ten years ago I worked at a vintage clothing resale store in Upper Haight at Ashbury, in San Francisco. I loved clothes and fashion, and fetish fashion—with all its shiny, tight fabrics and slightly sinister overtones—was one of my favorite genres. Perhaps this is where my corset fetish came from—to this day, I'm still not sure. Maybe it was the day when my gay male coworker, a sexy well-muscled drag queen who did the best Cher I've ever seen, wore a black patent corset and asked me to lace him up. It was around noon and the store was quiet, though he giggled, got on all fours behind the check-in area, and looked over his shoulder at me with a wicked, wicked smile. I was instantly flushed and excited, aroused. It got even more intense when, while I had both knees on his ass and was pulling the laces as tight as we could make them go, I looked up to see another, very attractive man in a business suit waiting to use the dressing rooms — and he'd been watching us with a devious smile the whole time.

It was just a matter of time before I stole my first corset from the store. My boyfriend at the time had no interest in fetish, corsets, or anything even remotely kinky — he thought people who did S/M and dressed in fetish clothes were weird and "kinda sick." At the store we received a new sale of vintage items, including a big, old-fashioned peach-colored corset, with about a million laces up the back and even up the sides. I stashed it in my bag when no one was looking, and hid it in my closet at home, when my boyfriend wasn't looking.

One night, he went out with the guys for beer and I stayed home to work on some artwork. But the minute I knew he was gone, I pulled the corset out from under my shoes and hatboxes and...admired it. I looked it over, closer now that I was alone with it. I wanted to see how it felt on my body; I was out of my clothes in a second, though I struggled to learn how the corset worked as I sweated, cursed, and wiggled into it. I hooked the front hooks, but they kept popping out as I tried to finish the bottom or top hooks; I was frustrated, but then once I got the hooks finished I had the back laces to contend with. I used my bedroom doorknob to tighten them — and then tighten them again. It was a wholly new sensation, being so tightly wrapped. I could barely breathe.

My figure looked amazing in the mirror, though my breathing was labored. I flopped back on my bed, lying back to relax and feel the sensations that flooded my body. The feeling of constriction somehow made my pussy feel hot, swollen, and alive. It was like a light switch flipped from "off" to "on" in my libido. For the first time, I had what I'd describe as an instant hard-on. Within a just few minutes of getting the corset on, I had to masturbate immediately to release. And once I came, off came the corset.

I grew up in the 1970s and '80s San Francisco Bay Area, a time and place when no one wore corsets — I don't think I actually saw a corset until I worked in Upper Haight. But what a joyful obsession and a terrific sex toy corsets are for me now; corsetry and tight-lacing is my fetish. I'm lucky to be in a such a city and to be surrounded with fetish-positive people (the kink-negative boyfriend is long gone). But as we'll see in the following pages, fetish isn't always easy and fun, though it is a delightful aspect of sexuality. Nowhere do our sexual imaginations become more devious or playful than in the world of fetish.

Unfortunately, until now, fetish for the most part has been stigmatized; sexually it's the last frontier. For the mainstream media it's right out there with circus freaks and criminals — and worse. Fetish is sensationalized when people want to sell books or boost ratings: Trot out the human ponies, look at the fat people. But most everyone has a fetish, and while sensationalizations are fun to watch, those promoting them often get their facts wrong and miss the point that lots of people have really hot sex with their fetishes and with lovers who share that fetish. No one's necessarily "sick" — they're just having more fun than most.

Take porn for instance. Many people see porn as a way to watch every twisted, bizarre fetish or activity you can imagine, when the truth is that if you take a look at porn, really look at what's out there, you'll find the selection is really limited and fetish porn usually sucks (and not in a good way). Porn doesn't even "get" fetish (actually, I think most porn doesn't even "get" sex, but that's another matter entirely). Smoking fetish is a good example; I never quite understood smoking fetish. I have a sex-worker friend who has a smoker for a client: They meet, she smokes in her underwear, and he watches and masturbates. He's her favorite client—he's polite, clean, never pushes her boundaries, and pays her well. I rented a smoking video once and watched a series of very bored women smoke while wearing porn underwear and berating the viewer for being a "sick fuck." (Hey, that's me!)

But then I stumbled across the films of Andrew Blake, an erotic photographer who very clearly has a smoking fetish—or if he doesn't, he's got a very sensual, sexy appreciation for it. In his films I watched gorgeous European models blow cigarette smoke into each other's mouths, between their legs, through the crotch of nylons, and just plain sit around looking extremely sexy while smoking. Smoking fetish made more sense to me now, but only because of this rare instance in which a filmmaker made the fetish come alive—he didn't stigmatize it like in the porn video as something "wrong." He got it, and so did I.

Hopefully this book will shine a sexier light on the world of sexual fetishes than has been done in the past. This book is written for the fetishist, for their lovers, and for anyone who wants to make a fetish into a sex toy. Or, to maximize a fetish, figure out if you have a fetish, how to talk about it with a lover, "come out" about your fetish, or find community—or just hot porn. Not every single fetish is included here, and if your fetish is not represented (or given as much attention as you'd like), I apologize, but know there are plenty of fetish-sex nuggets throughout these pages that can add a little something extra to your fetish pursuits. Enjoy.

—Violet Blue

Chapter 1
Guess My Fetish

Sure, it's good to have sex. But the world of sex is so much more than making a baby, cementing a relationship, or having a quick release—not that all of these things aren't excellent reasons for genital stimulation. Sex is as much in the brain as it is in the body, heart, and soul, and I'll argue that our sexual interests typically take forms far more interesting and unusual than what we read in *Cosmo* and *Men's Health*, and all the cultural stereotypes about what we're "supposed" to do in bed.

You can go on a date, but maybe what makes or breaks the first impression is her shoes. Making love to your boyfriend feels fantastic, but what if your ultimate orgasm could be achieved if you pretended you were asleep throughout the encounter? Or perhaps your relationship is great, but you have your best sexual encounters in front of your computer, imagining yourself being crushed underfoot by a three-story-tall goddess. Maybe you have a simple fantasy of receiving oral pleasure while wrapped in skintight rubber, or even dream of spending an hour on your hands and knees as a human animal being groomed and, of course, serviced for "breeding,"

Fetishes, from simple spankings to elaborate full-dress enactments, are where our sexual id comes out to play. Many people think of a fetish as something funny, crazy, sick, outrageous, fascinating, weird, interesting, or—better yet—hot. Maybe the idea of fetish makes you think of fetish fashion—shiny gothic outfits made of rubber or leather, tight-laced corsets or shiny buckles, much like what a dominatrix or Batman might wear. Thinking about fetish might make you imagine the fringes of sexuality cranked up to their craziest levels—facial bondage, giantesses, balloon sex, amputee fantasies, men pretending to be babies, women pretending to be ponies. Maybe the idea of all these things makes you uncomfortable. And quite possibly, when you think about these fetish ideas, you blush, excitedly revisiting the one thing that turns you on the most.

Imagine the possibilities of being able to play with sex in any way you can imagine. Then think about what happens when people who dislike sex imagine the same thing: The idea of fetish becomes a way of shaming any non-mainstream sexual interest. It's fun to think about the more far-flung sexual practices out there, but it's also important to know that everyone, no matter how "normal" they think their sex life is, has a fetish. And if your sexual interest, or fetish, is unusual or might be met with dismay (or worse) should your secret come out, it's essential to gain perspective on what your ideas of "good" and "bad" are when it comes to coming, and to learn how to mine your fantasies for all they are worth.

The truth is, when you look at cultural stereotypes of what constitutes "normal" sex, pretty much anything you do outside of heterosexual missionary intercourse can be considered "deviant," and in reality, everyone has a fetish of one kind or another—a position, eye or hair color, or body part.

This is the first book of its kind, an explanation of fetishes that doesn't negatively portray them as bizarre, deviant acts practiced only by a handful of people. That's because fetishists are not in a sexual minority, especially when you consider pop culture's widely accepted fetishes for big boobs and big dicks; even human ponies have numerous conventions, hold well-attended events, and publish magazines and newsgroups with hundreds of thousands of subscribers. In fact, fetish boutiques all over the world cater to their equestrian needs. Indeed, in many minds, people with fetishes occupy the freakish end of the gene pool when it comes to sex, and politely consider fetishes a place where people with far-out sexual tastes can get their needs satisfied.

What Is a Fetish?

Simply put, a fetish is placing greater meaning on something than it might have to someone else. When someone has a sexual fetish, an object, manner of dress, or specific scenario takes on a magical quality, has deeper value, and is often required for satisfying sexual release. The item or predicament becomes a reliable sex toy.

Fetish objects may include shoes, panties, a particularly meaningful item like a certain sex toy or garment, a brand of shoes (like Puma), corsets, balloons, bridles, messy foods, machines, sports bras, handcuffs, office chairs, bandages, piercings, hair, scars, tattoos, diapers, medical instruments, stuffed animals, uniforms, and much more. Fetishes for particular body parts are common, such as those for the neck, navel, breasts, anus, thighs, hands, and elbows. However, it's often more than just the item itself that sets the arousal switch to the "on" position; it's usually what's done with the item that does the trick. Fetish predicaments can include sniffing, being smothered, being "forced" to do something, bound or restrained, being punished with the item, humiliation around the item, being crushed by it, being rubbed and caressed by it, being "caught" with it, secretly enjoying the item, watching someone else take sexual satisfaction from it, having it withheld, watching it be crushed or destroyed, experiencing sensory deprivation or restriction in association with the fetish, or being regarded as a certain type of person, animal, or thing in association with the fetish.

Sensory fetishes include the smell of leather, rubber, undergarments, shoes, particularly scents such as perfume or bodily excretions; the look of certain fabrics or wet clothing; seeing one's self in a sexual situation or predicament; seeing others take pleasure with a fetish object; witnessing taboo or impossible sexual situations; watching pretty girls smoke, sneeze, or smear themselves with food, and more (seeing anything sexualized is possible on the Web, where photo and video manipulation is an art form). Sensory fetishes can also include restriction of one or all of the senses, or being forced to use a sense, such as tasting something fetishized, like a bodily fluid. Sensory fetishization can incorporate the feel of rubber, leather, silk, satin, sandpaper, or other material, in addition to binding and restriction, or even having bodily parts "inflated" with saline injections (which may induce as much visual and physical pleasure for the participant as for the observer). Aural fetishes typically center on the sounds of sex or masturbation but can also include coughing and sneezing.

Scenarios can incorporate the thrill of doing something in secret; being caught; getting away with something; touching something or someone; stealing a fetish object; being "bad" and punishment; humiliation, domination, or submission; feeling helpless or omnipotent; voyeurism; becoming something physically impossible (such as an animal, fantasy creature, alien, or baby); repetitive enactment of a particular fantasy; having sex with someone powerless (like a mannequin) or unconscious (sleep fetish); shaving or the act of being shaved; the fantasy of being tiny and inserted into orifices (and/or being crushed); wearing clothes of a different gender; undergoing embarrassing or frightening medical procedures (enemas, ob-gyn exams, prostate exams), and much more.

Fetish fashion has its own luxuriously naughty category in the vast world of sexual fetishes, and incorporates more interests than just wearing the right shoes. Leather, shiny rubber, PVC, plastics, liquid latex, corsets, stilettos and fantastically high heels, stockings, and more can be found in this highly sexualized realm of fashion. Fetishwear is a worldwide industry, especially in North America and Europe, and "fetish" often becomes synonymous with S/M and goth culture. Often, fetish events and S/M play parties are one and the same. It's not an inexpensive obsession, but if you've got the money, rubber, and corsets, hard-core human animal play can be explored to its furthest reaches. Fetish balls and conventions are typically high-fashion events with strict dress codes that embrace a wide variety of fetishes—and usually you can't even get in the door if you're not dressed according to code.

How Do I Know if I Have a Fetish, or Just an Interest in Something?

The lines between having an active sexual fetish and an interest in something blur to varying degrees. For instance, you might have a fantasy of being spanked by Anne, but you'd also like it if your other lover, Jenny, donned a rubber dress and fucked you with a strap-on. At the same time, for the past several years you've kept a secret panty collection from your old girlfriends and you occasionally masturbate with items from the collection. To top it all off, big tits drive you crazy, and you wouldn't dream of dating a girl with A-cups, and for some weird reason you come hard and fast when your mouth is forcibly stuffed full of titty—even better if you're spanked first. Meanwhile, you saw pictures on the Internet of a guy having sex with a balloon and it kinda turned you on. Quick quiz: Which one of these sexual interests is the fetish?

Strictly speaking, if this were you, dear and gentle reader, you would have a big-boob fetish, a panty fetish, along with mild spanking and smothering fetishes. The big breasts are number-one in the fetish food chain here because they are nearly *required* for satisfying sexual release. The panty collection is another, milder fetish, as it's a long-term interest and the panties are a constant supply of many happy masturbatory sessions. Spanking and breast smothering seem like nice additions and are constant interests, though on the fetish scale for you they're not needed on a regular basis for fantasy-induced orgasms. Balloon sex, rubber dresses, strap-on fucking, and dominant women are all interests, and should you discover them to be reliably exciting interests they may develop into fetishes, — i.e., something you'd like to see happen as a regular part of your sexual experiences. But often we live our whole lives with several mild fetishes, things we like to have in our sexual repertoires but are really just icing on the cupcake, not the whole bakery.

How Do You Get a Fetish?

No one gets hit on the head, like in the movies, and wakes up with a fetish. Clinical explanations about fetishes evolving from childhood experiences and Freudian experiences with parental nudity all reek with the same contrived stink as 1950s theories about homosexuality. Sometimes there is no rational explanation for having a particular fetish — though fetishists themselves are typically so articulate, if you asked them you'd likely have an interesting and articulate conversation about what, why, and how their fetish came about.

Some people have sexual interests that seem to have no explanation as to where they came from, or how they developed. A mummification fetishist who may love the restrictive feeling and become instantly aroused by the look and feel of wearing a tight rubber mummy bag may have no history with rubber in their past, have grown up in a modern household where no one wore bandages or wrapped outfits, and had no experience with mummy-bag imagery until their adult years. As with many fetishes, the fetish is something that instantly sexually "clicks" for them, and much of the confusion (and even anguish) around their fetish may stem from not being able to understand why this is, or where the feelings come from.

But fetishes don't just always "happen" to nice people. Sometimes a fetish can develop over a period of time, or after a few successful encounters; a spank-ee may not know or even have the desire to nurture a spanking fetish until they see sexy images of it, try it a few times, and decide they really like it *a lot*. Also, as with mild cultural fetishes like a predisposition for blondes, someone might decide to groom and cull and explore that part of their psyche until it becomes a fetish—dating only blondes for a year, or even the rest of their lives; masturbating to hot pictures of blondes; and gravitating toward blonde friends and acquaintances. (Note: A blondes-only hiring policy is illegal!)

Just as a fetish can be "discovered" and even pleasurably cultivated, in some cases it's possible to tone down your interest in a fetish, controlling your behavioral sexual interests and even changing them altogether. If your interest in panty theft disturbs you, perhaps buying used panties from Internet sources may adjust your behavior into something you find more acceptable (and you won't run up your girlfriend's panty bills). Or taken a step further, you can alternate actual panty enjoyment with Internet voyeurism until you feel okay about the adjustment levels of your sexual practices.

There seldom is a rational explanation as to why a particular person is attracted to a certain pair of shoes, wearing restrictive and beautiful corsets, watching women smoke in the nude, or likes to pop balloons during sex. We have many culturally accepted explanations as to why big boobs and huge cocks are fashionable sexual fetishes, but people with fetishes outside the norm are often stigmatized. This can be tough to cope with when you or your lover has a fetish and want to make it a shared sex toy.

Only Guys Have Fetishes, Right?

Fetishes do not discriminate based on gender, race, or class. The fetishes themselves do not choose to be good or bad, to be owned by men or women. There are female fetishists who eroticize the same objects in the same manner as do men, though we tend to see more of the male perspective on the Internet and in magazines because men are considered the primary consumers of pornography.

Fetishists surround us, and no one can even tell. People with fetishes are usually well aware of their fetish and have put quite a bit of thought into the who, what, where, why, and how of enjoying that fetish. The garden-variety fetishist is likely articulate, well-read, computer savvy, has theories about their fetishes, and even the least-savvy fetishist has a serious sense of self-control about the way they conduct their sex lives. Many live with the reality that they cannot share their fetish with their loved ones, so they discreetly set aside a time and place in their lives where they can find fulfilling release with their fetish, away from the risk of offending people they care about. Many fetishists visit professional fantasy-makers, such as dominatrixes, and have a healthy understanding of negotiation and boundaries (and if they don't, they learn the hard way, from pro dommes who won't let boundaries be crossed and typically do not engage in sex with clients as a rule). Most fetishists have healthy, happy sex lives with their lovers in the style of sex that their lovers prefer, though some partition off their sexual fetishes from their relationships. This can be isolating, but no one needs to feel lonely in a relationship, or feel confused about getting their needs met. This guide is for understanding and making the most of your—or your lover's—fetish, and learning that "normal" sex is *exactly* the kind of sex you enjoy.

Mother Superior
Thomas Roche

She was curled up on the edge of the sofa, him sprawled on the far side.

"I read that story you left out on the coffee table," she told him.

She never looked up from the electronic engineering textbook she was reading.

His face turned red. "You read it?"

"You said if you left anything out I could read it."

Of course he had. In fact, he had hoped she would read it—had *known* she probably would. But some part of him and thought she wouldn't—it was too much to hope for. Too easy. Too hot. His cock was already stirring.

"What did you think?" he asked, feigning only half-interest—not very successfully.

"A tender love story that speaks to the heart of the human condition," she said, still not looking up from her textbook. "I especially liked the part when I shoved my cock up your ass."

"Did you?" he gulped.

"Yes, very much. And when I spanked you. Do you really think you'd shoot that quickly? All over my school-girl skirt?"

He squirmed. "Um...I think I'd come, yes. I'd be rubbing against your thigh and everything."

"Tsk, tsk," she sighed, still not looking up. "All over that nice, pretty skirt. You'd probably leave a stain, you know."

"Yes," he said, his voice squeaking a little. "I guess I would."

"I'd *really* have to spank you, then," she mused.

He crossed his legs, struggling to reposition his painfully swelling cock.

"Of course, I don't even own a schoolgirl skirt. But if I had one, I think it would be very naughty of you to stain it. Of course, in the story, I reward you."

"Reward me?"

"Of course. You *want* my cock up your ass, don't you? A nice big, fat strap-on?"

He cleared his throat. "In the story," he said nervously.

"Oh," she said, eyes fixed on circuit diagrams. "Just in the story?"

He thought about it a minute, his heart pounding, his cock reaching full erection.

"No," he said. "Not *just* in the story."

"Hmmm," she said. "Would I have to be dressed as a schoolgirl?"

"No," he told her. "You...the schoolgirl outfit was just a fantasy."

"I see. A nun's outfit would be just fine, then? Nuns can give spankings, too. Schoolgirls usually *get* them."

"Um," he began. He had to squirm some more to get his cock out of its awkward position, tucked uncomfortably into the elastic of his shorts. "A nun?" He struggled with the words. "Um. That would be fine, yes."

She put down her textbook, spreading it on the side

table as she looked at him pointedly.

"Because, you know, that was part two of the story."

His brow furrowed. "Part two?"

She smiled, slowly running a hand down the front of her tight T-shirt. She wasn't wearing a bra, and her nipples were quite evidently hard, showing plainly through the thin cotton. Her panties were tight, too, and when she untucked her legs and spread them slightly, tucking one foot up on the couch and edging it toward him, he could see the moisture glistening on the thin fabric. Her smile broadened.

"Yes," she said. "Part two. Where you're the one dressed as a schoolgirl, and I'm your mean Mother Superior who spanks you and then fucks you in the ass when you come."

She had a rapturous look on her pinkening face, her arousal clearly growing as she spoke. She was positively glowing, and he could smell the scent of her sex even across the couch.

He looked puzzled as he readjusted his cock, striving to find a place where it didn't surge against his sweats. He finally found it, the head popping out of his shorts and almost reaching the waistband. "Part two?"

Her smile, now, was wicked, a mix of evil and tenderness that made his cock head pop, fully, out of the top of his sweats.

"Yes," she smiled. "Part two." She reached over and fished loose-leaf pages out of the back of her textbook.

"Would you care to read it?"

"Yes, Ma'am," he said breathlessly.

She gave a chuckle verging on a girlish giggle. She spread her legs a little more and cradled the precious sheets proudly.

"Then come over here and sit in my lap, little girl," she said with a wink. "Mother Superior has a story to tell."

"Yes, Ma'am," he repeated, and crawled toward her.

Chapter 2
Sexual Secrets

Living with a fetish is a bit like having a roommate in your sex life. Sometimes he comes home at the wrong time. Occasionally you have an extra guest at the sexual dinner table when you just want to have time alone with your girlfriend. The toilet seat gets left up—as in, sometimes you get unwanted downloads on your hard drive or your shoe-sucking porn collection is inadvertently left on the desktop. But then, this particular housemate also offers unlimited sexual satisfaction in a very specific, highly pleasurable way that no one has ever been able to—way better than a roommate that keeps the house clean, cooks your favorite lasagna, or watches the entire *Buffy* collection with you and cries at all the exact same times you do. But a fetish isn't a person, or a relationship, and having a fetish can be fun, confusing, sometimes lonely, sometimes irritating, extremely satisfying, even unintentionally hilarious, and it can teach you things about yourself. It can teach your lovers things about you, too—things that can bring you closer together.

Actually, the roommate analogy is a good one, but for people whose fetish doesn't make any sense in the context of their lives, or when the fetish involves things most might find distasteful, it's not very funny. This is when your fetish is an uninvited guest, and no amount of persuasion can make your guest leave. Sometimes you just have to learn to live with the strange and inexplicable fact that balloons make you wet and/or hard, that girls with missing limbs are your ultimate sexual fantasy, or that you'd be the happiest person on Earth if you could spend the rest of your life feeding your giant girlfriend until she's so fat she can't perform even basic bodily functions for herself, and this idea gets you off like nothing else. You don't understand why you feel this way, but you do, and when you sink into it you're at peace.

It's difficult to understand, and even more difficult to explain to people who don't know anything about fetish; or even more specifically that your fetish likely has online communities, porn portals, magazines, possibly even conventions, and support gatherings. You may not even know this, either—that living with a fetish is not a solo venture for the rest of your life, one in which you must enjoy your secret pleasures outside of your regular relationships. Some people might even feel so bad and confused about their fetish that they wonder if they're mentally ill, or somehow damaged. Even with the most seemingly benign fetish it can be a lonely feeling.

When your fetish makes you uncomfortable (and confusingly, aroused at the same time), you might worry that somewhere inside you lurks a bad person, a person who "deserves" something harmful. Even worse, you may feel you actually want your uncomfortable fetish to come true. Outrageous, physically impossible—and even illegal— fetishes are not uncommon yet can be extremely disturbing to contemplate. These fantasies are just that—fantasies—and there they will remain in the realm of imagination or in the safety of fantasy play with someone you absolutely trust. Remember, just because we have a fetish for an idea or scenario doesn't mean we wish it would really happen, on any level.

Conversely, living with a fetish represents freedom for many people to finally enjoy sex they way they like it, on their terms, and to finally give language to their true desires and the strength and power to ask for what they want. For all genders, this is a moment of personal power and liberation we were never given growing up, and having to experience sex in narrowly defined terms, by someone else's rules, never made sense to us anyway. It's the moment of "Ah!" where you find that one specific thing that really turns you on, maybe for the first time, and for a number of women it can be the moment of finally experiencing an actual orgasm. And then when you find a community of others like you, one in which you can joke, find comfort, even complain about how hard it is to find a decent amputee-fantasy porn site, well, you start to feel okay about the rest of your life, too. Things get a little easier.

Discovering that you have a fetish is a lot like the moment when you figure out you've been putting the wrong gas in your car, or that pizza is way better with pineapple, or that your cat was shredding your curtains because she was trying to tell you something all along.

Depending on the degree of your fetish and your self-determined levels of enjoyment, this moment of discovery can offer many things: realization, happiness, excitement at discovering a new sex toy, an explanation about your love of other people's scars, or even a moment of abject horror, shock, and surprise that something like this works for you.

Often it's a moment of instant arousal that seems to come from nowhere. Fetishists have described it as "a key turning in a lock," or "a light switch being flipped into the 'on' position." It's the instant turn-on, albeit a different turn-on than when a lover touches you in the right spot, or says the words you want to hear, or when you see a really hot babe do something sexy (though hopefully we'll combine your fetish with all of these things later!). For a mask fetishist, it could be an inexplicable desire to wear a mask and a feeling of being overcome with arousal so instant and powerful it must be satisfied on the spot — within reason, of course. As I've explained earlier, fetishists are not compulsives and understand restraint, consent, and proper time and place — even if developing this knowledge from early experiences with their fetish came from crossing boundaries and finding out the difficult way, as happens with young people figuring out their sexuality.

Of course, as wonderful, scary and exciting it can be to have a fetish epiphany, it can also be a moment of understanding and dread that you have a sexual secret, of sorts. And just how do you explain it, let alone share it, without making your sex partners run screaming from the room? Should you even tell anyone?

Fetishes and Relationships

For some people, their love for masturbating into Puma sneakers is a private thing, and they're just fine with keeping it that way. Others might feel really guilty about having a secret they hide from their lover. Many might feel so much love and affection for their partners that they want to share this really fun and highly specialized sex toy and have fun with it together. And for the single fetishist, it's tough to date within small communities and find people that you're compatible with beyond the shared fetish. Plus, dating can be a scary trial of disappointment, error, and hurt feelings and can be downright depressing enough to make you want to keep it a secret forever.

We determine our own levels of what's sexually healthy for us; no one else can do that. What is one culture's version of normal is another's idea of deviance; what's important to keep in mind are personal boundaries, people's feelings (and not hurting them), enjoying yourself within reason and limits of the law, consideration for others, and respect for other people's preferences and needs. By determining your own level of what's healthy for you—doing no harm to yourself or others, keeping your fetish from interfering with other parts of your life (like work, relationships, and friendships), not beating yourself up about it or blaming others for disappointing you in some way, and feeling okay about being a sexual person—you can enjoy your fetish as you would any other sex toy.

Are you ready to share your fetish? Ask yourself:
- Is your fetish going to be as fun if someone else knows about it?
- Would it be better kept as a masturbation toy?

25

- Is the content of your fetish of a potentially shocking nature? If so, is there a way to build up to it or test the waters?
- How far do you want to go? Actual enactment of your fetish, or just dirty talk while having sex?
- Would role-play be a good option? Or is that exactly what you want?
- Think about what you really want to do with your fetish and a lover in detail (I know, yum!). If you want to take the next step to talk about it, you'll need to be able to give them specifics on what to do, and how to do it.
- If you're met with rejection, can you handle it?
- Needless to say, never surprise a lover with your fetish.
- Can you live with it if you never get to enjoy your fetish with your lover?
- What if your lover reveals they have a fetish, too— possibly one you don't like?

We're made to enjoy sex, and we're engineered to share it. All too often, we know what we want but don't know how to get it. If you decide to share your fetish with your lover, it doesn't always mean that you'll be met with enthusiasm, or if you are, that your lover will be able to understand what they're supposed to do, how to do it, or what role they play in all of this. Opening up can be scary, and encountering shock, surprise, or distaste is even scarier. Start by learning how to talk about each other's desires (not just yours) and picking up tips for starting the conversation.

Whether it's a lighthearted panty-sniffing fetish or extreme adult baby role-play, sharing your fetish will bring you closer. It's a moment of discovering each other's sexiest secret wishes, and a chance to make them come true. Your pact to explore sexual adventures together can take you into exciting new territory, far away from your old sex routines, and can heat up any relationship. And in your relationship, your mutual willingness to try new things will take you both to the next level.

When you share a fetish, you're allowing each other into your own private worlds. Even if the fetish is owned by only one participant, you both get to play with it. Often our hottest fetish fantasies come from the places we visit in our heads when we masturbate, so it's important to know that in sharing this you both might feel emotionally exposed. You have to trust your partner to withhold judgment about your ability, performance, and (even scarier) your having a fetish in the first place. Confront your fears and your partner's by discussing the fetish together beforehand and establishing sexual communication. Coming out about your fetish might mark the beginning of a deeper level of trust in your relationship, and you might learn that your lover has a few secrets, a fetish, or an unrequited fantasy or two, as well.

Not everyone is going to feel vulnerable revealing a fetish or fantasy fuck scenario involving chocolate syrup and Easter Bunny costumes. Some will be empowered, most will feel finally free to truly express themselves sexually, and many others are just going to enjoy having unusual sex. It can be incredible to run wild with your fetish, whether in your head during sex or in real life, with an eager participant. And when a couple *can* play together, a once-secret love of human pony play just might make your relationship empowered by trust, energetically vibrant, and sexually alive. The intimacy and sexual closeness found in fetish play is intensely arousing for many people; this intimacy can be a very powerful aphrodisiac.

Does Your Lover Have a Fetish?

As the partner or lover of someone with a fetish, your moment of discovery might be filled with surprise, shock, anger, jealousy, confusion, awe, curiosity, arousal, excitement—and possibly even a sigh of relief to be able to finally share your *own* desires. Hopefully you'll see it as a newfound quest to understand your sweetie even more than you did before. Maybe you discovered something by accident, such as a stash of porn under a bed or in a computer folder. Perhaps you noticed a pattern of your lover lingering over certain objects or dwelling on certain scenarios. Maybe your partner saw a movie with a scene or read a story with something in it, and they just keep talking about it. Or, if you're lucky and your partner really loves and trusts you with their innermost sexual secrets, he or she told you about their fetish.

Whether it's something you just suspect, or something your partner laid out for you to react to and cope with, it's important to understand what he or she is going through, too. Ask questions—ask a lot of questions. But before you make any decisions about the relationship, or what kind of person your partner is, or whether you can trust him or her any longer, ask yourself these questions:

- Are you upset, angry, hurt, freaked out? Can you take a time-out to think about it before reacting?
- Does this change the way you see your partner as a person? If so, why?
- Do you have a fetish of your own, to even out the

playing field in your conversations? (It's okay if you don't.)

- Do you want to add the fetish to your sexual mix, or should it remain her or his private thing?
- Can you use this as a sex toy for yourself as well?
- How does this affect your trust, and are you willing to explain that to her or him?
- Would you rather the fetish be kept a fantasy, or are you interested in exploring new sexual possibilities?
- What do you need to know in order to feel okay about the fetish?
- Is there a way you can exploit your lover's fetish to the fullest, making *you* her or his fetish? Do you want to do that?

For many reasons, you may not want to try out the fetish, or you might want to make your lover happy but don't understand what to do, or what it means to you. Understanding your concerns and hesitations is essential; you'll need to have a constructive discussion about it, especially if you want to learn how to overcome fears that might hold one of you back. Plus, you'll want to figure out how to resolve what to do when one of you feels okay about it while the other doesn't. Remember — just because your lover told you about their fetish doesn't mean they feel okay about it,. You could be the one person they trust the most to help turn the fetish into a healthy sexual outlet rather than a lonely, confusing, guilt-filled solo pursuit. Or, if you've been handed this book with a smile of hope, you might learn how to set your concerns aside so that you can enjoy your lover's fetish purely for the pleasure of becoming their number-one fantasy fuck, and the one person who can get them off like no one else, ever.

If your lover wants to try something sexually that you're afraid of or unsure about, or feel morally at question with, it can bring up powerful feelings. Adding any new sexual behavior to a relationship can feel like a make-or-break situation, and sometimes it is. Asking to try styles of expressing sexual intimacy can push your relationship to higher levels, or it can bring up so many issues that it changes everything, forever. When sexual desires make someone feel insecure, unsure of their motivations, or the content of the fetish makes one of you uncomfortable, it can rock you to the core. This is especially true with fetishes related to degradation, fear, force, body manipulation, gender, age, or abuse. Remember that just because someone has a fetish for disturbing images or scenarios, it doesn't mean they want this to come true. Most likely their fetish is for the fantasy and nothing more.

How to Start Talking About the Fetish

No matter what, when someone wants to have sex, whether full-on fetish encounters in rubber and deprivation gear or a simple blowjob, one of you has to say "I want to." Many who are introducing a fetish to their shared sexual repertoire might receive a mixed reply—part interest, part hesitation. A few will be met with a reluctance to talk about it, and others might face outright refusal.

Talking about your fetish will be easier if you already talk about sex and experimentation in your relationship; it'll be frightening if you never talk about sex. Not everyone will feel comfortable discussing their sexual secrets, and you'll likely feel apprehensive about confessing your fantasies and desires, especially if you just learned about them yourself or have never talked about your fetish to anyone else before.

Telling your lover you want to try something new sexually can be stressful no matter what state your relationship is in with regard to sex. And if your fetish makes you uncomfortable, this is an understatement. In fact, even *thinking* about talking about sex is stressful sometimes! If you've never brought up the subject of sex with your partner, then it'll be a long-overdue conversation; it's a long-held belief that good, "right" sex just happens and without talking about it, the right partner for you will somehow magically "just know" exactly what to do to make you happy and satisfied. Considering that physically and mentally our sexuality is as unique to each of us as a fingerprint, nothing could be further from the truth.

If you're the one bringing up the fetish, reverse roles for a minute: If you don't normally talk about sex in your relationship and then suddenly one of you wants to, it can be a jarring experience that brings up a lot of questions—questions that *must* be asked and answered. Your lover may wonder if you've had sexual secrets all along. But it's very likely that this opening-up will provide your sweetie with an opportunity to finally be able to tell you what's on their mind about sex, too.

Before you confess your innermost sexual secrets, think about how you can bring up the subject in a way that feels safe. Perhaps you could watch a movie together that contains a scene pertaining to your fetish, giving you a convenient way to bring up the fetish in conversation later (during the movie is not a good time; it'll get glossed over as the movie plays, and you'll want more than a passing comment, no?). Another way might be to ask your sweetie what she or he thinks about sharing fantasies, while entwined in an intimate cuddle after your regular way of having sex. Another technique you can try is stating outright that you want to confess a sexual fantasy and that you want to hear one of your lover's, too—a fantasy trade. Tell them that you can have a conversation about it later; this will give both of you time to let the ideas settle in.

Think about things you can say to encourage your partner to hear you out, and ask them to suspend judgment until you can explain why your fetish is important to you. Especially stress how much fun you think the two of you can both have with your fetish—and how important their participation is to you. Be sure to reassure them that you wouldn't even bring up the idea unless you felt safe to tell them your deepest desires.

The most important thing to think through beforehand is how you are going to make your partner feel safe when you talk about it. It's essential to spell out how hot and sexy you think your lover is, and that this isn't a replacement for them, that you don't want it to replace the other kinds of sex you already have, and that the fetish does not compete with your lover in any way. Your lover needs to hear that they are still the absolute star of your show, in addition to the fact that you want to become more sexually intimate with them than you've ever been before, or with anyone else.

Sample Conversations and Outcomes

Before having your talk, think through possible scenarios and imagine how your lover might react, so that you'll be prepared to flow with whichever route the discussion takes. Rehearse what you'd like to say in your head before you actually have the conversation. Here are a few sample openers:

- "Wow, did you see that quick scene in *Secretary* where she wore the saddle and he put the carrot in her mouth? I thought that was kinda hot. What did you think?"
- "I read this short story with a scene in it that turned me on, but it was kind of unusual. Will you read it and tell me what you think?"
- "It would drive me crazy if you ever wore a rubber dress. Want to go to one of those stores and try one on so I can lust over you?"
- "Will you hate me if I want to try something kinky with you?"
- "I've never been in a relationship where we can talk about anything, like I feel I can with you. Want to trade sexual fantasies?"

When a Fetish Is Scary or Disturbing

Sometimes having a fetish is taboo enough to have life-changing consequences, and what we deem acceptable sexual interests varies from culture to individual. For instance, in San Francisco it's expected that a few week-ends a year you'll see men in leather-fetish outfits roaming around celebrating local parades and street fairs, even waiting in line for coffee at Starbucks in little more than chaps—whereas in a small conservative town in, say, Nevada, an arrest for indecent exposure would be the least of the leather-clad fetishists' worries. And while one par-ticularly open-minded sex partner may not understand your fascination with rubber gloves, they might be willing — or even excited — to pull on a pair and stoke you all over until you pass out from pleasure. Another lover may not understand this at all and might find it offensive. Though rubber gloves are not amputee porn, sex fantasies about sleeping or passed-out partners, or adult baby play — all things that lie *outside* what many people consider acceptable, or even quirky, fetishes.

When your fetish (or the fetish of a loved one) falls into a category that might be scary, disturbing, or even outright offensive, it's tough to cope with, let alone find people to talk to about it with who won't shame, judge, or condemn you. Again, having a sexual interest in something involving questionable consent, physically dangerous or impossible circumstances, or even illegal activities does not mean the person with the fetish (or fantasy) wants them to come true. However, it does mean the person finds a taboo, or aspect of it, sexually interesting to them, and this is something that can be constructively explored alone and with others.

If your lover has a fetish you find disturbing, suspend your judgment and ask them what's arousing about it — and how you can heighten the experience for them. You might find that "playing asleep" with your boyfriend is a total turn-on, or maybe it's only something you want to do once or twice a year. If the fetish upsets you, tell your lover as openly as you can and explain why, if possible.

Many fetishes exist only in the realm of fantasy. It is the *idea* that is most exciting and arousing to the fetishist, and visual stimuli (like online porn, real and fake) often fulfills the desire perfectly. If your lover has a fetish you find upsetting, don't be hard on them or think of them as a "bad" person; instead understand that he or she is simply a sexual person with a sexual imagination.

It's easy to feel out of control when it comes to things we don't understand, especially when they trigger strong feelings and sexual impulses, or sexual shame. Think about where your feelings of shame and confusion are coming from—stop giving someone else your power—and learn as much as you can about the fetish and how it makes you feel by asking yourself questions and checking in with yourself often.

Perhaps your discomfort doesn't come from an outside-the-norm fantasy, but instead raises upsetting questions about sexual orientation. Fetishes involving gender play can be as simple as a man masturbating in panties, or as ritualized as a woman undergoing a full transformation to effectively pass as a man. Neither means the fetishist is gay, transgender, or wants to become something they're not.

Still, gender-based fetishes can be frightening if you don't understand them or how you feel about them, and the feelings can be so strong that they challenge your ideas about your sexual identity in ways that make you feel uncomfortable. Many cross-dressing fetishists don't see it that way at all but simply use their fetish as another sex toy or masturbation aid. Meanwhile, others might feel so strongly that they embrace the challenges to their sexual identity, allowing the transformation to shape their sexual identities into configurations that are much more comfortable for them than their original manifestations. Either way, don't believe the *Silence of the Lambs* Hollywood-bullshit stereotypes about cross-dressers. It's exploitative hype, pure and simple.

Wearing the clothing and adopting the mannerisms of the opposite sex cannot make you into the opposite sex. It will not make you gay or lesbian, or change who you are attracted to or how you sexually identify. It also will not show you what it's really like to be the opposite sex. It doesn't mean you're transsexual or transgender, though for those individuals it might be the first step toward feeling comfortable with who they really are. If your lover is the one who's confused, explain that you aren't hiding anything; being a man and wearing panties during sex doesn't mean you want to be a woman, or for her to be a man. Light gender fetish play is just that.

Other common but often disturbing fetishes include role-play involving significant age differences and sexualized animal fantasies. These fantasies have playful cultural archetypes (stripper in a schoolgirl outfit, telling your lover to "bark like a dog!"), but these fetishes may be disturbing for people who confuse fantasy with reality. Role-playing in which one partner is much younger than the other, or is a dog, does not mean that either party truly eroticizes young people or wants to have sex with an animal. Those who molest children do so. People who harm animals do so. These people do not have anything to do with people who ask their girlfriends to pretend to be the older, sexually experienced baby-sitter, women dressing in school uniforms to play-act with their husbands, the man being pampered as an adult baby, or the boyfriend who likes to be bridled, saddled, and ridden around the apartment.

It's possible to feel okay as you begin the fetish play and afterward feel uncomfortable with the associations, memories of past abuse, or personal meanings the fantasy brings up. Sexual fetishes and fantasies are powerful because they have their roots in our subconscious and the oft-mysterious workings of our libido. If you find that your fetish play ignites memories or feelings that disturb you, read about taking steps toward sexual healing in Staci Haines's *Survivor's Guide to Sex,* or watch her video, *Sexual Healing.*

It's important to understand just what is appealing about these fetishes and role-play scenarios: Human animals and adult youth get to be "taken care of," and the feeling of not having to be in control is a blissful and incredibly arousing relief for many. Gender fetishes allow you to "try on" the other half, even if for just a short time. Read more about the ways these fetishes are fun and meaningful for the fetishist, and how to make these encounters even hotter in detailed sections in the rest of this book. Even if you decide it's not for you, you'll put this book down with a deeper understanding of your lover and yourself, and hopefully have a few new ideas of your own.

Chapter 3
Fetishes and Sex

Having a fetish usually means you have a preferred style of masturbation that works especially well for you, and presumes that most people who have fetishes enjoy them in relative solitude. Though this isn't always true, and many fetishes involve another person in one way or another, it's probably pretty safe to say that most fetishists spend a good amount of quality time with their fetish in privacy. In private, our fantasies can run willy-nilly through our masturbatory playgrounds, with no one to have to explain anything to, and wide-open vistas in which we can discover new ways to turn ourselves on.

Perhaps as a solo fetish practitioner you have a desire to make your fantasies become a bit (or a lot) more realistic. Maybe you'd like to see just how far you can take your fetish to make your masturbation sessions scorching; or you might simply want to get to know the whys, wheres, hows, and whats of your fetish to feel more at ease with yourself. For the soloist (if you will), all of your (private) world's the stage on which you can safely, comfortably explore your fetish.

One of the main things that hold many people back from being able to feel comfortable with their fantasies and fetishes is sexual shame, mainly shame surrounding masturbation. But masturbation is healthy, good for the blood flow to your genitals, good for your sexual imagination, great for learning more about yourself sexually, and can be a helpful tool for showing others how you sexually "tick." But lots of people learn to masturbate in quiet, hidden ways. We learn to lie about our masturbation habits so as not to look like "bad" people or hurt others we perceive might be upset or offended by this normal, healthy style of self-pleasure. And the things that we — everyone — fantasize about while masturbating are never to become polite dinner conversation, let alone something you might tell someone you care about the most. This is especially true when our fantasies and fetishes are far from the "accepted" versions of sexuality along the lines of Ken-and-Barbie, missionary-position, married-heterosexual (and accessory-free, I might add) porn.

Another issue that might compound your secrecy and hinder your fun masturbatory fetish adventures is the widespread notion that people in relationships should no longer, or shouldn't need to, masturbate. This fallacy turns your ability to show someone how you sexually tick into a ticking time bomb of sexual frustration — and even resentment when you can't or don't get your needs met by your partner. People in relationships can, should — and I'll even argue that they *need* — to masturbate, alone and with their lover. Our sexual private time is just as important as when we were single, and being a sexually healthy individual within your relationship keeps the relationship healthy, too. Being sexually self-reliant is realistic and complements — even fuels — an already great sex life. Partners who masturbate and enjoy private solo sex are not "cheating" on their lovers, though some people perceive it that way. They're taking care of — and doing something nice for — themselves. So stop feeling guilty already, and let's see how we can make those solo fetish wank sessions explosive.

To make your fetish masturbation sessions hotter than they already are, all you need is a little forethought, attention to details, and possibly a few online shopping excursions. First of all, think about your fetish and how it turns you on, and what you'd like to see happen with it. Often, adding a few touches here and there is all you need to make your fetish fantasy more realistic.

Pictures, movies, and visual examples of the fetish are typically the hallmark of how people enjoy their fetishes. Visuals might be a reliably traveled route for you, they might be a way for you to get started enjoying your fetish even more, or seeing your object of affection could be the next step in taking it to a better level. People with fetishes for things that are difficult to come by, rare items, situations that are difficult to create in real life (or even impossible, like giantess fetish) will be well-acquainted with images, illustrations, CGI, and videos, all typically found on the Internet. You may have favorite sites, galleries, and groups, and are always on the lookout for more, or are questing for images that take your fetish fantasy to the max — and I can assure you that somewhere it's out there.

The great thing about using images to enhance your fetish is that they allow you to sink deeply into your fantasy; porn is a great way for you to imagine that you're the boot slut, the human puppy, the one that's being smothered beneath a panty-clad ass. And with your hands free while you look at the screen, monitor, magazine, or book, you can (of course) touch yourself, and you can also feed your fantasy by incorporating an element of the fetish directly into your physical experience. So the boot slut can "force" themselves to worship an actual boot; the puppy can collar themselves, chew a bone, hump a pillow (substitute for a leg?), drink or eat from a bowl; the panty suffocator can even go so far as to order a pair of used panties online (see resources in the back of this book) and put them on a sex doll or ass-molded sex toy (again, see the resource section) and smother themselves while watching the on-screen action. Visuals alone let you "become" the person or thing onscreen that turns you on. But get a little creative—a little fetishy Martha Stewart, if you will—and you can create and improvise plenty of props to combine with visuals and make your masturbation sessions much more intense.

Think you'll feel silly? So what! You're not doing this for anyone but yourself. But maybe feeling silly (or even humiliated) while you stuff a pair of strange women's panties in your mouth and masturbate takes you a step further into the pleasure zone... And if this is the case, I highly recommend buying yourself a mirror large enough to see yourself while you play. Some people really get off on the humiliation aspect of their fetish—being seen doing the "forbidden" thing. A mirror reflects this state back at you very nicely; you can see just how "bad" you're being.

For many people, their fetish is their sex toy. For some, adding an actual, standard sex toy to the mix might crank up their arousal volume to eleven, just like the amps in *Spinal Tap*. For example, maybe the fetishist has a fantasy of being a pony that is bred with stallions: it's no problem to bring the masturbation session a step closer to the fantasy by donning "pony gear" and purchasing a dildo of appropriate size, with which she or he penetrates themselves with during the "breeding" encounter. Dildos, vibrators, and male-masturbation devices of all shapes and sizes can add a nice touch (literally) to any fetish fantasy. In fact, due to the particularly morbid nature of many male-masturbation devices, things like RealDolls (though expensive) can stand in nicely for necrophilia or sleepy-girl fetishes. In fact, many "pocket pussies" and limbless jack-off torsos sold under the guise of "sex with your favorite porn star body part" can add the only touch of realism you may ever need to fuel your amputee fantasy. Hey, I'm just pointing out the obvious here, folks...

Speaking of obvious, don't stick anything in your ass unless it has a flared end *and* is made for putting in your ass. Notice the "and"? A good number of sex-toy companies are just out to make a buck and produce unsafe sex toys. Most of the unsafe (read: trip to the ER) toys on the market are anal toys that don't have a stop at the end to keep them from being pulled involuntarily in the anus. Ditto for any other object, even if it's your fetish item: The anus convulses and contracts all by itself and loves to pull things inside. See Chapter 10, "Fetish Sex Rules," for more information.

That's not all I have to say about sex toys. I've deliberately kept S/M toys as part of a separate discussion about fetish masturbation. The fetish for rope is hot and sexy until you've imprisoned yourself and have to pee (and pee isn't your fetish), or worse...getting hurt and becoming unable to free yourself, being stuck in an actual emergency, being discovered (and that's not your fetish, either), or tying your bonds too tight and seriously injuring yourself. Not to mention the small but significant number of autoerotic deaths of people who bind their necks during masturbation. While you may be able to flog or spank yourself à la the film *Secretary*, putting yourself into bondage (handcuffs, ropes, restraints, silk scarves, etc.) is not at all recommended. Asphyxiation, while a not-uncommon fantasy, is extremely dangerous to attempt, especially alone, and is sadly fatal. Electrical play, too, has much room for error—like the error of accidental death—and should only be done by those who are experienced with electricity, or should be learned from an expert in electricity and S/M. Blindfolds are fine, as long as you're absolutely sure no one will discover you and that you're totally safe to go without your sight.

Use common sense when you play with asphyxiation, bondage, electricity, mummification, pain, or any sensation toy (see Chapter 11, "Resources," for further reading, websites, and information). Little clamps and clips can be used safely to intensify pinching sensations, though keep in mind that they hurt much more when you take them off, as the sensation rushes back to the previously clamped area. These items can be purchased in a sex-toy or S/M boutique, a hardware store, or even a stationery store, but they should always be tested on the soft flesh of your arm first—they can hurt worse than they look. Be wary of clips with teeth, which can puncture your skin and do more damage than you think. Clips and clamps can be placed on the fleshy parts of the body: breasts, nipples, stomach, thighs, labia, skin of the penis and testicles, even lips and earlobes. But don't leave them on for longer than your masturbation session.

Fetish and Partnered Sex

Many fetishes involve more than just the person with the fetish; they involve another person, even if the fetish centers on a body part, an act (like crushing or pouring raspberry syrup over a naked body), or a pair of smelly gym shorts. When you think about your fetish and turning it into a toy for two, this sounds like it makes sense; to play with the fetish, one performs the act, wears the item, or offers up the body part in question.

When the fetishist is into inanimate objects, imaginary creatures, impossible scenarios (like amputee fetish or scar fantasies), or a clandestine solo act (like theft), putting together a hot scene for two might require a little (or a lot) more creativity, imagination, and information to make things work—for both of you. Some people may not even know they have a fetish for certain objects, devices, or scenarios (and maybe you're trying to figure out if they do with the help of this book). Those who are aware make it easy to get the most out of the steamy sexual encounters you can have with a fetish. Of course, due to the very nature of sexual fetishes, details on sex with fetishes will be specific to the nuances of the fetish, but you can figure out a lot if you get at least a few details to start out with.

In any situation, however, the more information you both have about the fetish (suspected or known), how it's hot, how it can be made hotter and made to work for both of you, the better you can have fun with it. Before you explore the fetish with your partner, be sure to go over the following list of fetish questions together.

Questions to ask yourselves:
- What is the fetish?
- Is it a thing, a person, a body part, a feeling?
- What is the physical object that comprises the main part of the fetish?
- If there isn't an object, what's the most important part of the fetish?
- How does the fetish make the fetishist feel when they think about it?
- How does the object, scenario, part, or item make the nonfetishist feel?
- What is the main turn-on in regard to the fetish?
- Is there a particular time of day (or night) associated with this fetish?
- What does the fetishist like to do with the fetish?
- How does the fetishist like to imagine themselves involved with the fetish?
- How does the nonfetishist see themselves involved with the fetish? (If you're not sure, that's okay. This is to help you find out where you fit in.) Try a few guesses.
- If you're comfortable, the fetishist can explain how they like to masturbate in regard to the fetish.

Notice that I didn't include any questions about where the fetish comes from, early experiences with the fetish, or potentially disturbing uses of a fetish. That's because these topics are covered in the first two chapters, so if you skipped to this section first, skip yourself right back to the beginning of the book and find out more about these questions—and how to talk about them—before proceeding any further.

If you're uncomfortable just plunking down and going over these questions together, as many people might be, you can photocopy the list, answer the questions, and give them to your lover — or better yet, make two copies, write out your answers privately, and trade papers when you're through. This way, you'll have a foundation on which to base your fetish explorations together, and information on making the experience hot. Next, decide just how far each of you would like to take your first fetish scenario — and how realistic you'd like to make it.

As I mentioned in the preceding section on fetishes and masturbation, you can choose to enjoy the fetish primarily in the realm of your shared imaginations, or you can watch scenes in movies or read erotic stories to each other (from books or websites) that depict the fetish in action. This is a great way for nervous lovers to test the waters together; your fetish will be a vicarious thrill and you won't feel awkward in your Snoopy costume if it doesn't work out and he decides that it's just pictures of illustrated girl-Snoopys that turn his crank. Some fetishes will only involve images, photographs, or videos. This is a great opportunity for hand jobs or fun sexual positions. Also, fetishists who like having something rubbed on them can be disallowed to masturbate while you rub them with the object, and you can take your time masturbating them to orgasm. If the fetish centers mainly on images, like drawings or other impossible-to-become fetish fantasies, there are a number of ways you can include yourself in a fetish-sex session.

Playing With an Impossible Fetish

- Take control of the fetish. If it's on a computer, take control of the mouse; if it's in a movie, the remote control; if it's in a book, only you can turn the pages.

- Take control of your lover. Tie their hands so they can't masturbate while getting turned on looking at the fetish images.
- Let your lover have control of the images they look at but not control over their own genitals. That's right— you get them off while they look at the pictures, videos, or IKEA catalog. If you've ever had a fantasy of being an oral-sex slave, this is a great outlet for this fantasy as well.
- Get resourceful. Help them find more of what they like.

Sometimes just talking about the fetish and the fantasy it entails is enough for a hot bout of sex. That's right—good, old-fashioned dirty talk. You don't have to sound like a Discovery Channel narrator or a squealing porn star to make hot talk work; all you need to do is describe in detail a scenario involving the fetish. If you feel nervous about this, relax and remember that your lover is going to be concentrating on the content of your words, *not* the inflection or quality of your voice, and they'll be too excited to critique your performance. Plus, you can distract them with your hands, naked body, or fetish-related props (like your boob in their mouth, etc.). You can even simply describe exactly what you're both doing at that very moment—it's that easy. Try to let your mind to really sink into what it is you want to say, and feel free to keep talking to make up for figuring out what to say next; blabbermouths are great at this!

Tips for the Fetishist
- Tell them all about your fetish, or as much as you feel comfortable with. Focus on imparting constructive information that they can use to get you off.

Explain exactly what turns you on about your fetish so your lover can utilize the information to the utmost.

- While "in the moment," be sure to split your attention between your fetish and your lover. Err on the side of giving them more attention than you give the fetish, especially as you establish trust surrounding this new sexual activity.
- Don't be selfish; you can focus on yourself when you're alone.
- In situations where your lover is totally not sure about any of this but is willing to give it a try, make a show of getting off on what your sweetie does for you. Watch out for jealousy in regard to the fetish; remember, they might be worried that they now have to compete for your attention. Do everything you can to avoid having your lover feel threatened by your fetish.
- Trade sexual pleasure for your fetish and get your partner off in whatever way they like best: Just be aware that pleasing them first might make them feel like you're getting them "out of the way" so you can ignore them and enjoy yourself. There's nothing worse than lying back and staring at the ceiling through a session of cunnilingus knowing that someone's doing it out of "duty." Don't fall into a pattern of pleasing them first, in the middle, or last — instead, vary the pleasure you give them throughout your exchange.
- * Remember at all times that your fetish, when shared, is like any other sex toy for two. If it doesn't work, switch activities into something you know you both like.

- They are trying this out for you — and if they do it regularly, they're still doing this to make you happy. Always keep the compliments coming: Tell your lover how hot they look, how aroused they make you feel, and afterward tell them the things they did that made you see stars.
- Remember that you're not alone. Your lover wants to be there for you. And there are Internet support groups and message boards for virtually every fetish community, no matter how obscure.

Tips for Making a Lover's Fetish Hot

- Not sure about all of this? Never do anything you feel uncomfortable about or might feel bad about later? Know your limits and boundaries. If it's too strange or you still don't understand, say so.
- Ask yourself some hard questions and don't be afraid to answer them. Keep checking in with yourself as you explore your lover's fetish. Do you still like it? Are you seeing a side of your lover that upsets you? If it's not working for you, don't force it.
- Be totally up front about whether or not their fetish turns you on, and save yourself the resentment, detachment, and irritation you'll experience later. If it doesn't work for you at all, figure out and explain how you expect him or her to bring you to orgasm in exchange. Fair is fair!
- This is all about being open to new and unusual experiences and taking a playful approach to sex. It's like being able to play like a kid all over again, but between consenting adults.

- There is no reason for you to feel like you're the only one with a "weird" lover! There are tens, even hundreds of thousands of fetishists out there, possibly thousands who share your lover's fetish, and you can seek out web communities and message boards for support. You are one of *many* people whose lover has a fetish; you, fortunately, happen to be with an *honest* one.
- Get specific and discover how to playfully, erotically torture your lover with this prize piece of information about what gets them off the most! Ask questions: Do you rub the shoe all over your lover's body? Wear it? Make them eat from it or crush things with it?
- Try to persuade your lover to show you what happens when they masturbate with the fetish.
- Try to find elements of the fetish that excite or arouse you. You may discover you like having so much power and control over your lover's orgasm that it really turns you on to do something you might not think of as sexual. Or maybe you'll like the new sexual power and control you have over them.
- Push it as far as you can. Tease them, taunt them, rub it in their face, make their arousal as excruciating as possible before you give them what they want. Work it!
- Tease your lover by sending an email or slipping them a note explaining what you want to do with their fetish later. Then do it.
- Leave a fetish-related "present" hinting at what's to come later—tuck your panties in their pocket, give your lover a note with instructions, leave an erotic picture out in the open, or mark a story you want

them to read that includes the fetish.

- Surprise your lover with a new image, a new item for their collection, or a new "toy."
- If you live together, let them come home to discover their fantasy fetish scene waiting for their arrival. (But don't surprise them cold; let them know to expect something sexy when they come home, in case they have a bad day, or bring the boss home for dinner...)

Nurse's Duties
Thomas Roche

Marci put down the clipboard and smiled.

"Penis enlargement, huh? Sounds fun. How big did they make it?"

Brian had to suppress a laugh; Marci had this habit of mixing humor with her scenes. Normally this wasn't a thing he liked—but something about Marci's infectious enthusiasm made her perky goofiness more arousing than disconcerting.

Then again, maybe that was due—at least partially—to the skintight nurse's dress, decent at the hem by perhaps an inch, decent at the neck by—well, not decent at all, her ample tits spilling everywhere, white lace bra half-revealed between the low neckline and gapped buttons. The high heels and white stockings—the tops of which were maybe three inches below the hem of the dress—added to it all.

As did the fact that Brian was, indeed, experiencing penis enlargement at this very moment, underneath the pale blue hospital gown Marci had provided for him.

"I said, how big did they make it, soldier?"

Brian wasn't sure if the "soldier" meant they were now playing *M*A*S*H* nurse-patient or if it was just a convenient way to avoid using his name (Marci hated using names in the middle of scenes).

So he ignored the inexplicable soubriquet and said, "Fourteen inches."

Marci's eyes went wide, and she edged toward the hospital bed. "No kidding! Wouldn't that hurt?"

"Only if you do it right," snickered Brian.

Marci giggled and sat down on the edge of the bed. "You are so bad! You know, I've never seen one that big!"

He just smiled, and Marci peeled back the sheets. Her fingers trailed his thigh as she lifted the hospital gown, exposing his undeniably "enlarged" cock.

She looked for a moment then narrowed her eyes at him as her fingers trailed down to wrap gently around the shaft, making him shiver.

"That's not fourteen inches!" she said.

"No kidding," he said breathlessly. "I swear I'll sue that bastard doctor."

"No, don't do that," sighed Marci, leaning down as she stroked Brian's cock. "What's a few inches here and there?" Brian felt her warm breath on his cock for a moment before she extended her tongue and drew it slowly up the shaft. He moaned.

"Besides," she said, guiding his cock upright and rubbing it over her face. "He did make it *awfully* big. I doubt a girl my size could even take it."

"May as well find out..." began Brian, and then words were well beyond him as Marci's mouth descended over his cock, her tongue swirling on the underside as she swallowed him to the back of her throat, opening wide and deep-throating him slightly. He clawed at the hospital bed as pleasure suffused his body, and when Marci's body began to bob up and down rhythmically, he moaned louder and lifted his hips to meet the thrusts of her mouth. The little nurse's cap was so well pinned into place that it stayed there no matter what she did.

She teased him, gently, bringing him close and then backing off, tonguing his balls so that he cooled down—and he understood that she wasn't just going to get him off, she was going to fuck him.

"It is *awfully* big," she sighed as she crawled onto the bed, spreading her legs over him. "I'm not sure I can handle it."

"Oh, you can handle it," he grunted.

The front of her nurse's dress rode up, revealing that she wasn't wearing panties underneath. She slid on top of him, spread, and thrust his cock inside her, groaning.

"Oh, soldier," she whimpered. "It's too big!"

Then she began to fuck him rhythmically, pumping her hips back and forth as she drove his cock deep into her. She kissed him deeply as she fucked him, and the rattling of the hospital bed spurred her on to greater strength in her thrusts. The violent motion popped buttons on her dress, and she began to fall out of it, finally ripping the thing off and discarding it, wearing nothing but the white bra, garter belt and G-string as she fucked him. She cried out in orgasm, gripping him between her thighs, the hat still perched flawlessly atop her head as she came with great mewling groans.

He came an instant later, letting himself go deep inside her as she fucked herself on top of him.

"What do you know," she said breathlessly. "Turns out I *can* handle it."

"Nursing school must have paid off," he said, and pulled her down hard against him.

Chapter 4
The Heart of Fetish: Role-Play

One way to look at fetishes and fetish sex is to see them as boiled-down versions of sexual fantasies: an erotic fantasy stripped down to its essential element. Granted, as an element it might be an event, predicament, or object with no discernable context in which to place a fantasy, but that doesn't mean it can't be made into a fantasy or scene easily shared by two.

On the other hand, some fetishes are entire scenes unto themselves; whereas one person might verge on orgasm from the sight of medical instruments, the instruments can easily be put into the context of a medical-fetish scene. Indeed, some people might fetishize exactly that— medical scenes, with only a few particular elements and a loose script, or maybe they just wish a few specific things happened to them in a medical context.

When you share a fetish with a lover you'll be making a sexual fantasy come true for at least one of you — though I want to encourage you to incorporate elements the non-fetishist will enjoy, too. Everyone has sexy fantasies, has imagined anonymous sexual encounters, or even fantasized about everyday situations becoming sexual, such as work-related scenarios. If either of you has ever fantasized about pretending to be anything other than who you are in your daily, ordinary life, then you're ready to take the first step into making a fetish fantasy come true. All it involves is a little sexual role-play — or a lot, if it turns both of you on.

When you're not in what you consider your typical sexual roles, you're basically introducing an entirely new situation to your regular lovemaking routine. This can be as simple as adding a fetish-related detail to certain sex acts. For instance, you might introduce a blindfold, a pair of rubber gloves, high heels, or a nursing bra; as long as it's specific to the fetish, you're on the right track. Starting small and working your way up to the "ultimate fetish fantasy" is a really good idea if you or your lover is nervous about any aspect of fetish. If it's a scenario involving role-play, lovers who think being in character is more nerve-wracking than arousing might prefer a simple prop much more than the pressure of wearing an outfit and behaving differently. Figure out what makes the non-fetishist's participation erotically interesting for them, and make sure you're absolutely sure who's in charge of the encounter before you begin (especially if your scenario involves role reversals).

There is no "right" way to play with fetishes or roles. You don't need to worry about what anyone thinks or how any "experts" do it. Because fetishes are so unique to each person, simply enjoying it and having a satisfying encounter makes you the expert in your situation. You don't need to play by anyone's rules except your own. But if details outside the fetish, such as wearing the perfect outfit, make it all that much hotter, or a fake French accent makes it funnier, then don't hesitate to pull out all the stops. Yes, fetishes can be silly and hot at the same time. You can have fun and be a dork while erotically torturing your panty fetishist—and it may surprise you that a little bit of whimsy makes you more creative, and the scene that much more intense for your lover.

It's a good rule that for your first fetish-play encounter you should start out simple, even if you're both experienced with an aspect of fetish or BDSM. Even seasoned pony trainers will want to slowly ease into breaking in their new (even if totally experienced) pony girl; you'll learn more about what your lover likes, and it's a great way to savor what could turn out to be an unforgettable first time. Go slow—slower than you think you need to.

For complete first-timers, dirty talk can be a great way to dip your toes into the fetish pool. See if playing around with verbalizing during sex is even for you; if it's not, then now you'll know. Fetish play doesn't have to involve talking, but many scenarios will require some kind of verbal communication. If you're not used to talking during sex, try describing what you know about the fetish object or predicament, or what it would look like to play with the fetish (this can be imaginary, or you can describe what's actually happening). Tell your lover what you're feeling, especially if you're aroused.

Turn up the heat if you're playing a role: Tell the point of view of your character or role, such as "I'm a really naughty shoe-sniffer. I've been a sneak all my life and now you've caught me. I hope you don't punish me by making me smell your shoes." Of course, this is essentially telling your lover what to do, but that's the point. The person with the shoes can improvise, saying, "I can't believe I caught you smelling my shoes! I think that's really dirty and you're in a lot of trouble. I've had a really long day and I'm shocked to find you like this in my closet. I can only think of one thing to do, which is to make you sniff my shoes. You must touch yourself while you do so, but you may not have an orgasm until I say so, and you're going to make this worth my while by huffing every shoe in this closet." Or you can even use your true feelings at that very moment to make your role authentic: "I've never caught a shoe-sniffer before. Why don't you tell me how you think you should be punished?"

When you begin to take fetish play beyond merely the idea of the fetish and start to add details, events for a scene, or even costumes, it's important to make sure you're both clear about each other's expectations. He might want to be a panty thief, hoping to be caught and roughly punished for being in a "stranger's" bedroom, while you may think he wants you to model panties for him, or have panties rubbed on him while he masturbates—two very different perspectives and outcomes.

Know Your Roles: A Quiz

To get things clear before you dive into a fetish scene, copy the following questions and answer them separately, then show each other your answers; circle as many as apply and feel free to fill in your own responses.

My ideal fetish scene includes:
• Punishment

- Humiliation
- Teasing
- Doing whatever I want with the item, body part, or person
- Watching you interact with my fetish item or scenario
- Being something I'm not in my everyday life
- Conflict with authority
- Getting caught
- Being made to do something naughty
- Sex!

In a fetish scene, I hope to:
- Be sexually "used" by you
- Do what I want with my fetish
- Have you in total control of the fetish
- Get spanked or whipped
- Have my way with you
- Spank or whip you
- Lose control
- Call all the shots when it comes to the fetish

I'd like to be:
- In charge
- Helpless
- Someone who gets overpowered
- A submissive that turns the tables
- Equal
- The subject of some kind of sensory deprivation

My fetish involves:
- Oral sex
- Doggie style
- Anal sex

- Bondage
- Restraint
- Pain
- Messy play
- Smothering
- Images and fantasies in my head
- Body modification
- Animal fantasies
- Specific clothing, fabrics or gear
- Kinky sex (specify)

I want our fetish scene to happen in:
- Bed
- Our imaginations
- Public, such as a bar, restaurant, dance club
- A different room in the house than we usually have sex (specify)
- A hotel room
- A sex club
- A dungeon
- I have a certain place in mind (specify)

Ideally, clothing would include:
- Uniforms, at least for one of us
- Bandages
- Everyday clothes
- It doesn't matter as long as it includes... (specify)
- Clothing like our roles would wear
- Realistic costumes
- Nothing!
- Sexy lingerie
- Very fancy clothing
- Bondage gear

- Rubber, leather, PVC, other
- Gloves, shoes, a mask, corset, stockings, panties
- Animal accessories
- Adult baby gear

For me, the most important thing in the scene will be:
- Outfits (specify)
- Believability
- Being seen in public
- Getting in your pants
- Being in charge
- Your submission
- You fighting against me
- Not being in control
- You being forceful
- A particular sex act (specify)
- Spanking, whipping
- Sensory deprivation, such as blindfolding
- Restraint/bondage
- Humiliation
- Your fake limp/scars/neck brace

All of this makes me feel:
- Nervous
- Aroused
- Scared
- Afraid of what you'll think
- Ridiculous, but willing
- Excited, but unsure
- Like we're getting really intimate
- Like we're going on a sexual adventure together

The worst thing that could happen is:
- We'll be too scared to go all the way
- I'll be afraid I'll hurt you
- We'll get the giggles
- We'll have a clothing malfunction
- We'll decide that we don't like it
- It might be emotionally intense
- I'll disappoint you in some way
- You'll think I look/sound/act like an idiot
- We like it so much we do it again
- We give up and just have really hot sex instead
- We really make each other's fantasies come true
- We get raspberry syrup on the drapes/cat/inflatable St. Bernard

Okay, So Now What Do We Do?

Sex play with roles or desired actions requires context. As in, sure you're in the CHP uniform, but what are you *doing* as a California highway patrolman? Context for your fetish means that circumstances and events create the support for your role. A man can play a doctor, but he's just going to check your chart and leave unless the patient reveals that the bandages on her private areas are too tight—putting the doctor in a position of power and giving him a task, something to do.

Generally, context falls into two categories: someone being active and someone receiving or reacting to the person's actions, to varying degrees. One person takes the lead, takes control, acts, calls the shots, initiates the sex play, or is in control of everything. The recipient receives the action, follows the leader, lets the other person make the decisions about what happens first (or next), is submissive, or watches the scene unfold around them.

When you let the other person take control, you are not necessarily submissive. When you make a decision about what you both will do next, you are not necessarily dominant. But for some people, being in a submissive role is a turn-on, while others will find that taking charge gives them an erotic charge.

Developing your roles and giving them context gives your encounter meaning. A spanking is ordinary (or even silly) if you do it for no reason at all out of the blue and then you go on as if nothing happened (unless that's specifically your fetish, of course). But it can be sublime when you make it a fetish-tinged punishment and someone *forces* it to happen because someone else behaved badly (and they have a spanking-punishment fetish). Then, if all goes well the whole thing turns you both on to the point of ridiculousness, until the one in charge has to have their way with the spank-ee and everyone gets off the way they like it. That's a fetish tucked neatly into a successful and satisfying context.

A particular fetish item or predicament may be all that's involved. But then what happens? One of you has to do *something* with that object or scenario.

Being in control means you're in charge, and that can be to whatever degree you find comfortable, or what makes the most sense for the scenario. You may find yourself drawn to just being in charge of the sexual part of the fetish, calling the shots step-by-step, a little or a lot. You might be attracted to being in total verbal and psychological control, telling your lover to perform for you, rub your feet, give you head, or bend over. This model of dominance, sans pain or physical punishment, makes running a fetish scene simple to control in length, level of comfort, and even what type of activity you do (and don't) want to have happen. In some cases, you might even just adopt the role in your head, and not act on it but let it give you direction or inspiration for your fetish encounter. Of course, some control roles work well as submissive roles (especially in overpowering fetishes), and vice-versa, but here are a couple of lists to give you ideas.

Sample Control Roles: animal trainer, baby-sitter, boss, biker, celebrity or movie star, clergy, coach, criminal mastermind, daddy or mommy, doctor, dominatrix, football captain, gender-swap, general, headmistress, innocent jailer, kidnapper, nurse, older sibling, "pervert," pimp, police, master, millionaire, mistress, role from TV or movies, sex-worker client, sex worker, teacher, yourself (such as in daily life or role at work)

Does it sound better for you if you're not in control of the fetish? When you want to give up control, it doesn't mean you have to be a masochist. You might get a thrill out of being objectified with or by the fetish. You could be the silent handmaiden administering to your fetishist's erotic needs, in any costume or role that works best, or you can be a sex toy that gets used and discarded. That is, until you're needed for further use.

Sample Receptive Roles: altar boy/girl, butler, cheerleader, criminal, gender-swap, groupie, housewife, human pet (pony, dog, cat), "innocent" passerby, maid, masseuse, military subordinate, nurse, patient, prostitute, schoolgirl/boy, secretary, sex worker client, slave, submissive (as yourself or your real-life work role), unsuspecting husband, victim

Make It Happen

A little planning is essential, but spontaneity will still the rule the day when you're in role. Even if you're allergic to planning out a sexual encounter, or worry that even the tiniest agenda will take all the fun out of it, you at the very least need to know what your goal is and how to get there. You can always pretend to play mistress and sissy maid, fall out of role when you crack up after he asks for a feminine hygiene product, and still wind up tearing each other's clothes off (apron and all) for an orgasmic finish. All you need is a good strategy for getting started.

First, when will this go down? Give yourself a time frame long enough for the fun to run its course; an hour is a good idea. You'll want to be able to take your time, especially if all goes well. And as I mentioned earlier, make a point of going slow and making every bit last as long as possible so your fetish scene will be effective and have a lasting impression. Make sure there will be no interruptions—that your roommates are gone, the kids are away—and turn off your phone, IM, and anything else that likes to snag your attention. You don't want any distractions or interruptions to derail your adventure, and no one wants to risk having to explain their private sex lives to anyone.

If your scene might get loud, perhaps with yelling, barking, or the popcorn sounds of spanking or whipping, be sure to close your windows and doors, that the neighbors are away, or have a cover story ready in case someone "checks in" on you. Give yourself plenty of time to relax afterward as well. Stock up with plenty of water, any sex toys you might like, suitable porn, lube, towels, and props. Have yummy snacks and beverages waiting afterward as well—if your scene is successful it'll feel good to recharge, and if things don't go as planned, you'll have some nourishment to help you both center and regroup. These things are also nice to have if things bomb. Comfort food and drink and maybe even a movie to watch while you get your heads back together are always a nice landing, regardless of the outcome.

Surprise scenes should be planned out *very* carefully, and your lover must always have some indication of what's coming. What if you deck your apartment out like the set of *Star Trek*, apply your Klingon makeup, and she comes home upset and exhausted from an awful day at work? Let her know you want to plan a fantasy surprise, and give her an indication of which role-play scenario you have in mind. Like, "Want to meet me in the Holodeck when you get home?"

When planning a day in advance, provide a few time-frame examples to choose from, such as Wednesday, Thursday, or Friday evening. It's also okay to give an assigned date and time to come over or meet at a certain place—if you're in a dominant role, you can "tell" your lover to do it, or else! Tell your panty fetishist to meet you at a certain café, in his business suit for a surprise job interview. You will of course be wearing the appropriate panties, flashed at appropriate times. Then adjourn to your "office." Some surprise scenes will take careful negotiation, especially if they involve something in public, force or implied violence, or other people.

The Main Event: What Happens in Your Scene

One of the most important things you'll want to decide ahead of time is what your encounter will center on. Because even if it's an object that's the fetish, your encounter will be built around what happens with that object. You can have props or be totally naked, in a rented castle or your bathtub—extra details are nice, but it's *what happens* that counts. The event is the turning point in your scene or communication that changes everything. Chances are good you already know what this event is, and that's why you picked up this book—to make it happen, or to make it more intense.

If the location of your role-play is what's hot, such as when you have a public or semi-public scene, the event occurs when you show up. If it's a dressing fetish (covered in detail in the next chapter), then the event could be when you get dressed, the ritual of dressing and being watched (or assisted), when you see each other in the outfit or garments, or when you undress. If it's an object (or body part), then it's what is done with the object and how it feeds a particular feeling about the fetishist's relationship with the object.

For "power over" or sexual-coercion scenes, events can include:
- Talking your way out of something
- Not turning the fetishist in for their misdeeds in exchange for sex, or a demonstration of some kind, like a striptease
- Offering sex in exchange for goods or services
- Sex for a coveted job or career advance
- Getting out of punishments or jail time
- Bribery
- Settling a bill on the spot

With goals such as spanking or punishments, the event can be:
- Getting caught doing something forbidden

- Being a "bad" animal
- Acting sassy
- Being a slut
- Failing to do a chore or follow instructions
- A punishment for a transgression that never occurred

Other events can be psychological, such as:
- A learning experience, where one person asks for sexual instruction, or is convinced they need it
- Capture
- Getting picked up by a stranger
- Being a victim
- Slavery
- Embarrassment, humiliation
- Part of routine examinations
- Petting, grooming and playing with (as in with pets and animals)
- Being the "special" groupie, little girl/boy
- Doing something so taboo it's silent and secret

Make your atmosphere reflect your fetish scenario. Be creative and make over the room where you'll have your encounter just a little bit (or a lot), and it'll add that extra layer of validity and realism to your encounter. Of course, if your scene takes place in an ordinary room in your house such as a closet, lingerie drawer, kitchen, bathroom, or garage, you're all set and ready to go.

Practically anything can be improvised at home. For instance, your bedroom can be transformed into any setting you need. For a doctor's office or nurse's exam room, cover a nightstand with white paper towels and an array of instruments and exam items. These can include bandages, sex toys, rubber gloves, lubricant, washcloths, and items you don't plan on using but look good anyway. Use a shiny silver butter knife as a tongue depressor, and a butt plug as an anal thermometer. Neaten your bed into an exam table and cover it with a white sheet; get a cheap one at a thrift store if need be. Lead your sexy patient (victim) into the exam room when it's his turn.

Don't fret when you realize you've started the scene; it often feels like there's no turning back, but that feeling will ebb away when you take it slow. Take a minute to give your role some thought: Something in the role attracted you, or playing it for him turns you on, so something in that role resonates inside you. What is it? You're going to be nervous no matter what, so base your actions and reactions on that nervousness. Does that make you even more eager to please, or will you use it to overcompensate with your stern demeanor?

Keep reminding yourself about what you're doing and you'll feel less nervous every time you do so. Motivation is why you're there, even if you're just slathering yourself with chocolate sauce and sitting in a cheesecake. Relish it, and take your time. Your main goal is arousal and sex for all, and for you both to have a great time getting off in a new, exciting way. Your motives will always be sexual, though sexually different than the role or persona you're used to being with this person (though not likely too different than you'd like to be).

Say, for instance, you've been asked to be a sexy teacher who spanks the naughty schoolboy, and you don't usually do that. You'll likely discover that once you put on your teacher outfit you realize that part of you gets an erotic charge out of erotically dominating your boyfriend. If you're still uncertain but are willing to play along with the sexual fun and games, you can tap into your eagerness to serve up your lover's hottest sexual encounter—their fetish—on a silver platter. Give them what they want because you know how much it means, and how much it turns them on. And don't forget: There's nothing wrong with allowing yourself to really get into it, especially if you find it makes sex exciting.

Job Interview
Thomas Roche

"You've got quite an impressive resume, Miss Clark."

"Thank you, Mr. Williams."

"What I think is most interesting is that you wrote it in narrative form."

"Yes, Sir. It seemed to convey the full breadth of my experience better that way."

Mr. Williams paged through the papers on his desk. "I especially liked the way your last manager, Mr. Lorentz, enforced office discipline. Perhaps you could summarize that for me."

Miss Clark blushed. She plucked nervously at the buttons of her white blouse—which were unfastened to the point where the top of her lacy white bra was revealed.

"It's all in my resume, Sir," she said.

"Yes, it is," said Mr. Williams. "Fourteen pages of it. I'm a busy man, Miss Clark. I skimmed the high points. But perhaps you could summarize."

"Spankings, Sir."

"Specifically?"

"If I, um..." Miss Clark searched for the words. "If I stepped out of line, Sir. Mr. Lorentz would spank me."

"Yes, I see that. Over his knee or over the desk?"

"It depended, Sir. If I was a few minutes late getting

back from lunch, or if he caught me daydreaming at my desk, that was an over-the-knee offense. But once I stapled a revenue report instead of three-hole drilling it. That was taken much more seriously."

Williams leafed through the pages of Miss Clark's resume. "I see he bent you over his desk, bound your wrists to the corners and your ankles to the legs..."

"Actually, Sir, they were eyebolts. Mr. Lorentz had them installed in the floor."

"I see. And then he gave you quite a time of it, didn't he?"

"Yes, Sir. He started with the paddle, of course, but before long he used his flogger."

"A very heavy flogger, by your own admission."

Miss Clark's face was, by now, deep crimson.

"Yes, Sir."

"And at this point he had removed your panties with his letter opener?"

"Yes, Sir. And lifted my skirt."

"Must have been quite a temptation for him, having a pretty ass like yours all exposed and vulnerable, ripe and red from a well-deserved beating."

Miss Clark's breath came short as she squirmed uncomfortably in her chair.

"Yes, Sir. If you read on you'll see he yielded to that temptation."

Mr. Williams's eyes fixed pointedly on Miss Clark's face; a tiny smile played across the corner of his mouth. "I'd rather you tell me what happened, Miss Clark."

"Well, Sir," said Miss Clark, her voice at once small with humility and husky with excitement, "he fucked me. After teaching me a good and proper lesson, of course."

"He laid pipe in that fine ass of yours, didn't he?"

Miss Clark's eyes lowered; she could not meet her prospective employer's gaze.

Breathlessly: "Yes, Sir. That, too. After fucking me soundly the...the usual way."

"And did you learn your lesson?"

Miss Clark was breathing hard, her lips trembling. "Oh, yes, Sir. I never stapled again."

"We enforce office discipline in a similar way here, Miss Clark. Do you think you could 'fit in' here?"

Shivering, all over: "I think so, Sir."

"Look at the floor, Miss Clark. At the edge of my desk."

Miss Clark had already noticed them: eyebolts, set into the floor right where the big oak desk terminated.

"Let's find out if you can learn a new lesson from me, shall we?"

Miss Clark stood, pushed her chair back. "Yes, Sir," she said.

The oak desk was clean except for a phone, which Miss Clark obediently placed on the floor, and a few papers, which Mr. Williams tucked into his top drawer. Within moments she was bent over the front of the desk, her ass in the air, her tight skirt pulling taut as she spread her legs. Mr. Williams reached into his bottom drawer and produced a set of ropes, which he used to swiftly bind the interviewee to the hidden eyebolts in the corners of his desk. The ropes pulled taut, and Miss Clark whimpered slightly.

He reached back into the lower drawer and came out holding a handful of implements that made Miss Clark shudder and squirm with anticipation. Mr. Williams came around the desk, knelt down, and forced Miss Clark's ankles still wider apart, forcing her to hang, suspended, off the edge of the desk. Thick, padded leather restraints buckled tightly around her ankles and padlocked to the eyebolts. Mr. Williams set first the paddle and then the flogger alongside Miss Clark on the desk; the touch of the flogger's strands against her belly where her blouse had pulled up was enough to send a pulse deep down inside her pussy.

Mr. Williams's hand traveled slowly up the back of Miss Clark's thigh; he slipped his hand under the crotch of her thong and briefly felt her pussy, entering her with two fingers to establish just how much she enjoyed her work.

He then roughly yanked her short skirt up over her ass, and produced a letter opener — not the knife-shaped kind, but the safety sort, marked LETTER OPENER, which worked with a razor. It proved even better than the other kind at slicing through the straps of the miniscule thong Miss Clark wore; her panties fell, shredded, between her parted ankles.

Mr. Williams picked up the paddle.

The first blow made her jerk against the bonds and moan. Mr. Williams then punished her with a series of rapid blows, alternating from cheek to pale cheek, turning them rosy in minutes as she whimpered and ground her hips against the edge of the desk. Soon her pussy was glistening, her body squirming with every blow he gave her. When he seized the flogger, Miss Clark let out a cry that was halfway between dismay and ecstasy. The whirl of the flogger laid hot red stripes across her cheeks and upper thighs, bringing a shriek from her as Mr. Williams increased the power of each blow.

After a dozen strokes, his cock stood hard in his suit pants. He reached for his belt buckle, and the sound of it rattling made the squirming Miss Clark push her ass higher up into the air and strive to spread her legs wider.

His cock parted her pussy lips and she gasped. He drove into her with an easy thrust, filling her cunt in an instant. As he began to fuck her, she pulled harder against the bonds, straining to push herself onto her prospective employer — but he had bound her well, and all she could really do was stretch there, bent over the desk, and take each savage thrust of his cock as he penetrated her again and again.

She came with a bestial moan and then a long, luxurious sigh. Mr. Williams fucked her harder until he cried out and left the hot spurt of his come deep inside her, withdrawing from her wriggling body only after he'd fully satisfied himself.

"Excellent, Miss Clark," said Williams as he ran his fingers over the rising welts on her exposed behind. "You can start Monday morning."

"Th — thank you, Sir," whimpered Miss Clark.

Beautiful, thought Williams as he stroked his wife's reddened ass. Beautiful that a woman like her, a lawyer, well schooled, sophisticated, in charge, never a secretary in her life, could describe a fantasy in such delicious detail and that the two of them could see it through to its logical conclusion — her, fucked, over the edge of his big oak desk, bound and spread and vulnerable.

He was hardly finished with this scene — she most definitely would start Monday, albeit Monday night, when the two of them got home from work.

But then, in their world, even midnight could be Monday morning. And there was plenty of office discipline to enforce. She wouldn't even have to staple the reports. He felt confident he could always find something to punish her for.

Chapter 5
Fetish Dressing

What we wear speaks volumes about us. It can convey a mood, such as the choice of a skirt versus pants for a dinner party, or the decision to wear something sexy and revealing when going out to a club with friends. A tight shirt says, *I want to play* more than a conservative choice (like a turtleneck), which would communicate to passersby, *I'm just here for a drink*. Sometimes we dress just for comfort, as when putting on a pair of familiar, well-worn shoes for a run to the store, or a different kind of comfort, as when a meaningful item is chosen for a special occasion. Regardless, no matter what you decide to throw on, it's always a conscious choice of some kind, even if you're the kind of person who considers yourself an "I don't care, just want to be comfortable," T-shirt-and-jeans type.

But chances are good that because you're reading this book, you're not the "anything goes, no reason" type of dresser (unless you're reading this to understand someone else's choices). But taking a minute to consider the more pedestrian choices we make when sliding into our favorite leather jacket, comfiest gloves, or sexiest heels can open a window into understanding the world of fetish dressing.

Fetish dressing is when something worn on the body takes on a greater, more erotic and sensual meaning. The eroticism and meaning might come from the item itself, the ritual of putting it on or taking it off, or the type of fabric from which it's made. It could even be the manner of procuring the garment itself that gives the erotic rush—custommade items, a special shopping trip, the suspense or erotic rush from finding and bringing the item home.

Taking pleasure in what you wear is something that appeals to the sensualist in all of us—no matter if it's a leather glove or an intricate rubber costume. The thrill may come from being seen in the garment. Masturbating in the item. Feeling like something other than your ordinary self while wearing the item. Identifying strongly with what the garment says about you to others who see you in it. The physical feeling the garment creates, or just the smell, feel, taste, and sound of the fabric. It may be one, a few or all of these things that turn dressing into fetish dressing; perhaps it's the entire sensory ball of wax. And for those who like to see and be seen in their fetishwear, it's as much about the sensuality of the experience wearing the item(s) as it is attending parties and events in full fetish attire.

Fetish dressing is only the delicious finishing touch for some fetish and role-play experiences. For many, what's key is the entire fetish experience; the manner of dress is the main course, rather than the finishing touch on a scene or an added bit of realism that makes the medical scene that much more visceral. In many situations the scenario and the fetish dress involved are so dependent on each other that the full-on fetish experience is only fulfilling with the trappings and ritual of dress and final look of everyone involved for it all to come together. Fetish dressers exist on a spectrum of enjoyment, from the mild to wild, and their tastes and preferences for what they like to do and when may vary with moods, seasons, ideas and, of course, shopping trips.

That's not to say that some fetish dressers are all over the map with their practices and tastes. Some people know exactly what they like, when they like it and how — and would prefer never to stray from their routine. A favorite pair of rubber underpants (and all the care, cleaning, maintenance, and ritual of wearing them) might be the one thing they love the most and prefer to play with — you can keep your leather horsie gear to yourselves, thank you very much.

In fact, it's a misnomer to think that if one person is into rubber encasement and mummification suits, she'll be into rubber nurse outfits as well. Sure, she might fetishize the rubber aspect, but in fetish dress, unless the person is an all-around rubber fan, dressing fetishes will fall into a few neat categories — which is why medical and human animal fetishes, even through they involve ritualistic fetish styles of dress, are in another chapter. This chapter delves into the fun, folly, heat, and practicality of fetish and fetish fashion dressing. Typically, it's what's thought of when people say "fetish" in reference to clothing; goth style, S/M clothing, leather, rubber, PVC, latex, and everything you might see when attending a fetish dress event or party, or on a trip to a fetish dresser's closet (or dungeon).

If we were to peek into the worldwide fetish-dressing closet, what might we find?

Fabrics and materials such as: leather, rubber, PVC, latex, silk, satin, lace, spandex, metal, fake fur, plastics, shower curtain material, stiff cotton, crepe, canvas and more. In some instances your fetish experience might focus on the material; when the fetish is the garment itself you might not care what it's made of as long as it's a (panty, glove, corset, etc.). Typically, the material and garment are closely tied in significance, such as "the perfect leather bustier" or "my rubber tiger outfit."

Common fetishwear items (in fetish fabrics) may include: gloves, dresses, masks, shoes, heels, boots, corsets and neck corsets, body harnesses, bras, panties, lingerie, and restrictive or revealing skirts. Hobble and pencil skirts create an amazing silhouette (especially when topped with a corset), but make walking difficult, which might be part of the thrill of wearing the item. Period items like burlesque wear and fifties clothing also might be fetishized, in addition to uniforms, subculture "uniforms" (like leather daddy styles), and collars or cuffs. Also hoods (like "gimp" hoods), which cover the entire head and may have holes for eyes, nose, and mouth (or not) and may have D-rings for bondage or control scenarios, or a variety of other options.

Corsets and Tight-Lacing

A corset is a close-fitting undergarment frequently hooked in front and laced in the back, with boning, or stays that run top to bottom within the garment creating a cage for the midsection. It can cover from above the bust to below the hips, and garters can be attached. The old-fashioned Victorian corset has seen some (literally) breathtaking updates in the past 60 years, with resurgence in the underground fetish communities of the 1950s, to the present-day punk, goth, cyber, neo-Victorian and haute couture fashion revivals. The feel of being laced, the restriction of motion, and the hourglass shape the corset gives are powerful elements to a corset fetishist. Some may like to be corseted, see them being worn by others, or undergo corset training, where a corset is worn for extended periods, changing the permanent shape of the waistline. Corsets may be found in stores ranging from the mall-lingerie variety such as Victoria's Secret and Frederick's of Hollywood where you can find them for less than $100, all the way to custom boutiques where an off-the-rack model will cost around $500-$1,000, and custom-made corsets even more. Unless you're crafty or enjoy thrift-store and vintage-clothing-store corsets (where you can find real corsetry bargains), this can become an expensive fetish, especially if you like to collect the garments.

Corsets and tight-lacing can elicit a variety of feelings, from lust or excitement to resentment at reminders of women's struggles for equality or symbols of financial decadence. Corset enthusiasts are a very articulate and refined culture and likely have a lot to say about how and why they enjoy corsets and promote corset appreciation. Not all corset enthusiasts are "into" fetish, and not all fetish-loving corset wearers are "into" S/M, or corset training, and a few see them as symbols of oppression. In fact, some corset lovers who enjoy corsets as an integral part of their role-play — from Renfaire to Victorian vampire scenes — see the symbolism as an important detail in their fetish fantasyland.

But are corsets healthy to wear, especially for waist training? Historically women wore corsets practically every waking minute, as tightly laced as possible, and it was common for them to carry foul-smelling salts in case they fainted from restricted breathing. Fortunately, these days are past, but as with any tight garment, from corsets to cock rings, use your head. Only wear your corset at its tightest for as long as it is comfortable, or if you are waist training, follow your instructions to the letter. Tight-lacing on its own is not unhealthy; some people have trained themselves to wear a corset tightly for nearly 24 hours at a time. Of course, this is like being a top athlete in your field; it must be trained for carefully, and if you have health problems tight-lacing can exacerbate issues you may already have, especially those related to circulation or internal organs. Never bind yourself tightly in a corset with broken or cheap parts. If your corset feels good for up to an hour, you've found a comfortable fit that can be worn for extended periods; just the same, once you have a corset on, it will take your body about 15-20 minutes to arrange itself and adjust to the fit.

Corsets come in a variety of shapes and styles. How yours looks will depend on what you want it to do. Do you want it to be short (waist only), underbust, overbust, or half-bust? Do you want your waist to be hourglass, stemwaist, ice-cone, or waspwaist? How tight will you want it to go? And the bottom: Do you want it to be more like a girdle, long, short, hip length, or bottom length? And what about fabric or color? Sometimes fabrics determine what kind of corset can be made. Corsets are not easy to simply walk in and buy, unless you're just getting started — if so, buy a cheap and simple style from a lingerie retailer to see if it's even for you, before you invest time and money into a garment you may or may not even like.

A good corset has to fit our true measurements, making ordering corsets by mail a tricky situation; though for many of us, online corset shopping is our best option for selection and price. Very carefully follow the measurement instructions on the site you order from, and call the retailer if you have any doubts or questions about your order. And don't worry — corset sellers are used to customers who ask a lot of questions, and selling corsets to male customers is a routine transaction; according to the European Corset Society, male customers comprise half of all online corset sales.

Take good care of your corset and it will last you a lifetime. When purchasing your corset, ask the manufacturer for washing and care instructions; either way, never put your corset in a washing machine. Dry cleaners are typically your best option, with gentle hand washing in lukewarm water as a second choice. For all leathers, PVC, satins, and brocades, dry clean only; still, for these and all other fabrics consult an online fabric-care guide to be absolutely sure you can handwash your canvas camouflage with PVC-finish waist-cincher. Never wring it out or iron; dry flat between two towels with compression.

Gloves

People with a glove fetish might eroticize the look of gloves, the way they feel coming on or off, or enjoy being touched by someone wearing gloves. Each individual will have a preference for fabrics, but common materials for glove fetishists include satin, rubber, lace, and leather. For some, it's the sensation of slipping into and touching the world through a second skin of sorts; for others, it's being on the strangely anonymous yet intense receiving end of being touched by this fetishistic surrogate skin. Often, in addition to the material the gloves are made from, the actions of the glove-wearer contribute to the eroticism of the fetish as much as the gloves themselves. Refined glove fetishists will know their glove size and have collections for different moods; conversely glove fetishists on the receiving end may have a particular size hand and glove style they prefer. Gloves may also represent power and authority over someone; they are formal, and may signify an impersonal barrier that is the center of a dominant and submissive exchange. Some may like to masturbate with gloves on for an impersonal feeling, or as with rubber and latex gloves that heighten sensation and heat exchange, might enjoy the intense sensation on the genitals that gloves can produce.

Panties

Panty fetish has become so common in pinups and soft-core and hard-core porn that it's almost a cultural fetish that can be lumped in with big-breasted blondes and big penises. However, a panty lover is certainly not your garden-variety fetishist. More than just a gender-specific item of clothing, panties hold a special reverence for many people, making this fetish one of the most intense around; especially because it's common in people who typically don't think of themselves as fetishists.

Looking up skirts, getting glimpses, touching, smelling, being smothered, having them stuffed in the mouth like a gag, stealing and masturbating with panties can all be exciting for panty fetishists.

Panties bring immense pleasure to those with this fetish, and often the fetish plays on the notion of garments not meant to be eroticized; the forbidden, a girl's necessity, the mystery under the skirt, the part closest to a woman's genitals. Color, fabric, cut, and style are all particular factors for the panty fetishist, and enjoyment can express itself in the form of seeing, smelling, touching, masturbating with, stealing, wearing or purchasing panties. Panties can be used or new, freshly washed or very dirty, sometimes even better if they're still on the wearer.

Shoes

Shoe fetishists typically have a particular type of shoe that they fetishize, and may collect them to look at or masturbate with, get aroused when another person wears them, may want you to do something with the shoes while they masturbate (such as put a shoe in their mouth or step on them with the shoes), may want to have your regular style of sex while one of you is shoe-clad, or might just get turned on when you wear a certain pair of your own shoes. And we're not just talking about stripper heels here — shoe fetishists can lose it over mules, stinky slippers, Pumas, Manolos, and that big shoe fetish subculture, boots. A shoe fetish is not a foot fetish, but it never hurts to ask your fetishist if they like feet as well. A man who gets off wearing women's shoes isn't necessarily a cross-dresser, nor is a woman who get an erotic charge from wearing men's boots.

Less common fetishwear items include:

- Dildopants and dildopanties, where a built-in or inflatable dildo is part of the garment, either for vaginal or anal penetration (or both). These may also be molded to create a "cameltoe" or show the shapes and folds of the vulva, or for men might have a penis and testicles sheath, or one and not the other.
- Open nipple bras, typically molded to shape the breasts in a particular way, such as a "torpedo" style.
- Any molded latex items created specifically to show the topography of the body or to form the body into a new shape, like nipple bras, panties, cock/ball shaping items, latex wigs, and latex face masks.
- Pod and diving suits, made of rubber, latex or neoprene, often intended for submersion in liquid. These are full-body encasement suits, might be inflatable, and will have breathing apparatus specific to the fetishist's fantasy.
- Straitjackets, standard issue, vintage, or made of fetish fabrics.
- Rainwear, mackintoshes, and capes.
- Gas masks, respirators, and rebreathers; these look impressive and scary, feel intense, and control breathing. They are becoming more popular.
- Vac, or vacuum beds. Sort of like getting in a giant Ziploc sandwich bag and having all the air taken out, with a variety of respiration options.
- Total enclosure mummification, meaning the entire body is wrapped or sealed in a fetish material, such as rubber mummy suits, or wrapped in plastic

wrap. This is complete submersion into a material with absolute restriction of movement; holes may be left or created for genital, anal or nipple access. Facial and breathing options are open to the fetishist's desires.

- Animal suits, covered in the next chapter, can be as simple as a tail and pair of ears bought at the Halloween store, but in less common fetish instances can be elaborate rubber full-body, molded, and highly styled, masked affairs.

- Chastity belts. Homemade, bought at an S/M store, retro or vintage, simple or sinister—each limits male or female genital access to whoever installed the device, or has keys to the lock. While called belts, they're usually more like G-string-style underwear as if made by industrial designers, and may have onboard insertables such as butt plugs, vibrators, or restrictive cock cages.

- Inflatable garments can be full-body suits that blow up around the wearer, or might inflate to compress the wearer. Inflatables may also be specific use garments, such as hobble skirts or straitjackets, facial hoods, masks, or female suits that inflate to a female shape from head to toe. They may also be insertable inflatables (or include insertables within the garment) that fit into vaginal, anal or oral cavities. Not to be confused with actual body part inflation fetishes (see Chapter 9, "About the Body").

- Sleepsacks and body bondage bags, made from a variety of materials, fall into the mummification category also.

- Beds, sheets, and sleeping items made from fetish materials, such as rubber or leather sheets.

Female Latex-Mask Fetish

Female latex-mask fetish dressing — or masking — is male-to-female transformation into a mannequin, doll, or cartoon/cosplay character using a rubber (latex) mask that's very similar to a bondage hood. Masking is most popular in Japan and Europe, and involves rubber fetish, cross-dressing, and sometimes sissification or forced feminization. Because many practitioners combine the mask with tight-fitting corsets, rubber girdles, and layered clothing, there is an element of restriction, sensory deprivation, or bondage. Masks are often sold with accompanying torsos.

John Willie's *Bizarre Magazine* (Taschen) features forced feminization using masks from as early as the 1940s; most mask stories involve submissive women being masked and transformed into passive "living statues" for their master's viewing pleasure, though today the primary practitioners are male-to-female cross-dressers. The masks and torsos are crafted to create an essentially uncanny doll-like, hyper-feminine quality. The masker possesses an intense desire to transform into the ultimate sex object: perfect, blemish-free, stylized, mute, pretty — and usually pretty stacked. Zentai usually gets lumped into the masking fetish, though this Japanese fetish subculture edges away from feminization and into full-body encasement suits (like leotards), usually made from spandex or other shiny stretchy material.

Cosplay

Literally a contraction of "costume" and "play," cosplay is both a noun and verb: Cosplay is the act of dressing up like cartoon and gaming characters, and it's the act of live-action role-playing (or LARP-ing) as the characters.

Cosplay is typically a nonsexual pursuit, though there are plenty of sexually active cosplayers to make up for being in the minority. It's considered primarily a Japanese pastime, as it comes from Japan and many of the characters portrayed are from Japanese cartoons, live-action TV shows, pop bands, hentai, and manga. Cosplay is an extensive subculture unto itself, with conventions, costume contests, huge online communities, cosplay cafés and amusement parks (in Japan), and more. There is a sexy, gothic Lolita fascination in the sexualized aspects of cosplay, and an overlap into masking.

Dressing and Wearing

Once you have your garment in hand there is a world of sensual, delightful, and erotic tension-building ways for you to proceed. Maybe you're the type who just likes to get in the thing and play, no funny business standing between you and the act of wearing your fetish outfit or item. For instance, getting into the corset might be a dreadful pain in the ass, full of struggle and sweat and nearly pulled muscles, but once you have it on — pow! It's like an instant aphrodisiac, your waspy waist and the feeling of constriction conspiring to make you so erotically charged and turned on that you just can't wait a moment longer to get yourself off.

But chances are good that you might be the type of person who relishes the slow transformation, or savors the slow moments of pulling on those favored, those most erotic rubber opera gloves. Perhaps you drain every sensual moment you can out of the very act of donning your fetish outfit, making every deeply arousing minute last as long as possible. You stop to admire yourself, take stock of your situation: the smell, the feel, the sound of everything you do while getting dressed. Your solitude is your personal erotic ritual. Here, dressing is one of the ultimate erotic pleasures you can imagine, and you revisit these moments like your finest masturbation fantasies. In fact, they may be one and the same.

Dressing may not be an act of solo sensuality; you may fantasize or enjoy having another person involved in your dressing ritual. Imagining—or actually experiencing—someone watch you dress, transform, or get ready might be one of the headiest erotic experiences you can summon in your cabinet of fantasy. Or do you require, or desire, an assistant? A slave, handmaid, dominant, owner, personal tailor, slutty seamstress, corset wench, or loving partner in fetish bliss? Sometimes it's even more fun when you have help, an extra pair of hands or eyes, and in some situations, help is absolutely required (whether from a practical or safety standpoint).

You might find yourself on the other side of the act of dressing: the one who assists. Here your role is to help and thoughtfully aid in the deep eroticism involved in dressing, whether you're helping your lover slip into shoes or spending an hour slowly wrapping very inch of them up in pallet wrap. As you participate in this incredibly tactile sensory experience, it's also your job to participate in the reverence your partner places in their fetish garment. Inhale the scent of fabrics, enjoy the feel of the corset's stiff boning, sink deep into the weight of the rubber hood as you pull it over their face. Do their stunningly perfect boots, once in place and laced up, deserve a kiss? Think about the mood you set with your actions. Are you there to serve your lover's pleasure and beauty, or are you Pygmalion, turning them into a living erotic treasure? Perhaps your lover would get instantly aroused if you spent a long time blacking those boots, or shining the rubber catsuit *while* they wore it? Remember, the main essence of the fantasy you're creating is the fetishwear, and the person wearing it is the central figure of the erotic encounter. It's not merely the Lucite heels he puts on to wobble across your bedroom; it's the entire act of what it takes to be *him* in those amazing shoes.

Is the act, or rather art, of getting dressed just the beginning for you? Now you can choose from a variety of ways to enjoy your dressed-up self. You can play with your lover, admire yourself, sink into the sensuality of how it feels to be in your favorite fetish mode, enact a private (or shared) fantasy...or you can take your fetish out for real, not imaginary, eyes to admire and see you the way you are in your fetish form. Because taking your fetish outside of your private space might involve other people, be sure not to involve anyone in seeing something they may find offensive, or might turn them into nonconsenting participants in your own erotic enjoyment. It's not only not cool, but it may also be illegal depending on what you're doing and wearing. It's not just young eyes you'll want to avoid the risk of encountering; no one should be forced into a situation they don't want to be in. Be wary of what you show when you go from house to fetish event, or if you want to wear your garment out and about, either be absolutely sure it can effectively "pass" as a high-fashion—if a little extreme— garment, or can easily be hidden or obscured. Wearing rubber under your everyday clothes—or even just something to remind you for your fetish—can make for unforgettable (secret) thrills.

Fabrics and Feelings

The smell of brand-new leather—or the familiar scent of a particular leather jacket and the sexual thrill it brings when you touch the leather and inhale, deep. The tautness of rubber, its shine, the smell, and rituals of care it requires. The surface of your fetish heels, and the tingle they give you. The rough brocade of your fuck-corset. Often, our fetishes center squarely on the materials from which they're made. And the two biggest corners of those worlds are the realms of rubber (and PVC/latex), and leather.

Leather

The term "leather fetish" means different things to different fetishists and might mean something completely different in the gay bars of San Francisco than in the fashion boutiques of another city. But no matter what your leather fetish says about how you identify sexually—whether you're into S/M or motorcycles, or just the fabric—leather is home base for many fetishists. Foremost, leather is a second skin and layer of protection. It provides warmth and comfort; it's primarily used in commercial garments for fashion and because of its rugged protective qualities in motorcycle trousers and western chaps. It's easy to come by: Leather pants, gloves, skirts, dresses, and jackets of many styles are available in almost any boutique or department store. Thankfully, despite its mainstreaming, leather is also associated with rough sex and BDSM culture. Here it appears in the form of fetish garments, straps, bindings, whips, hoods, corsets, and all sorts of yummy suggestive clothing.

Leather-care instructions:
- Use a high-quality stain and water repellent. Apply right after you purchase your leather garment
- Use a good leather lotion and a soft cloth to clean the garment
- Don't use shoe or boot polish on leather items
- Heavy or sharp objects in pockets will stretch and dent leather
- Don't put stickers or adhesive on your leather
- Blot stains with a soft cloth
- Wipe sweat off ASAP; the salt will dry out your leather, which can lead to cracks
- Allow leather to dry naturally; never put it in the dryer
- Store leather in a way that will maintain its shape
- Don't store in heat, damp, or cool areas; leather will dry and crack in heat and mold in dampness
- Store leather garments away from sunlight

Rubber

Rubber fetishists eroticize the smell, feel, and look of rubber garments, gear, and rubber isolation suits, masks, and more. The rubber is worn by the fetishist or put on their lover, and might be sexualized in dozens of creative ways, including bondage, inflation (filling with air), and isolation, where the senses are taken away by masks, breathing is through tubes, and the entire body is encased in layers of specially made tight rubber garments and mummy bags. Some just think wearing or seeing a rubber dress, rubber corset, or tight-fitting shiny material is really arousing.

Latex rubber has many qualities that distinguish it as a

sensualist's fetish. It has a unique fragrance often described as sweet, like vanilla. In this way latex fetish is similar to leather, which also has its own distinctive smell linked to sexual connotations. Unlike leather, latex can be more like a second skin than any other material, and absolutely seamless. Latex can be molded or cast from genitalia and seamlessly attached to garments, sheaths, and insertables. Thin latex, when skintight, transmits the sensation of touch in a most amazing way, hence its success in use for condoms, and it's very exciting to wear something so thin yet impermeable as a garment. Latex alone has the ability to faithfully transmit the sense of touch, heat, and cold, and some even claim there is often an amplification effect.

Also, it sounds cool. Rubber, when walking, moving about, robing, or disrobing makes a unique sound. It snaps, rustles, and crinkles when the loose material contacts itself. Undoubtedly the sound of rubber is an attraction to many latex lovers. It also looks amazing, and carries a sheen like no other material on earth: Many of us love it simply because it's so shiny.

PVC is not rubber or latex but a type of plastic. Real PVC fabric is actually difficult to find, and most of the fabric sold as PVC is really PU (polyurethane). A good rule in telling the difference is that PU is stretchy while PVC is not; PVC is not sold with Lycra or other stretch backing because PVC cracks when stretched. It usually has a cotton or nylon backing with little or no stretch. Both PVC and PU clean up nicely with Windex.

To slip into rubber:
- Visit a specialty shop and have an experienced salesperson help you into your first garment.
- Theories conflict on whether to use powder (talc or

cornstarch) or silicone rubber-garment lubricant to slide into your rubber outfit. Talc has been linked in medical studies to cervical cancer, so keep that in mind and avoid vaginal contact with talcum powders. Some complain that cornstarch turns to sludge inside a wet rubber garment. Others swear by the tactile sensation silicone liquid provides; yet some companies insist some types of silicone lubricant weaken rubber and latex garments, causing them to tear. Always defer to the manufacturer's recommendations.

- Many people swear that shaving body hair is not only necessary but increases the erotic skin contact and heightens the sensation of wearing rubber. Experiment with what you feel most comfortable with. Read more about body shaving in Chapter 7, "Cross-dressing and Sissies."

- When pulling on a rubber item, gather it like a sock or stocking and release the gathers as you slide the garment over your body part; never grab, tug or pull hard on the fabric or it will rip.

- Getting out of your garment usually means inverting the garment as it comes off your body, turning it inside out.

- When trying on rubber outfits, always wear under-wear.

- Always follow the rubber care instructions as per the individual garment maker.

Going Out: Parties and Events

So, you're all dressed up, but do you have anywhere to go? Fetish fashion is a huge worldwide industry, especially in North America and Europe, and the sexuality inherent in "fetish" blends with S/M practices and gothic style — and it's common to see fetish events that are also S/M play parties. Fetish balls and conventions are typically high-fashion events with strict dress codes that embrace a wide variety of fetishes — as long as the attendees dress to the nines. But dressing for fetish events may not always be what you think — it's important to review an event's dress code before you even think of going shopping. Most fetish events have strict rules about what's okay and what's not; your business suit might be the hottest fetish item you have in your closet, and the biggest turn-on for you and your lover, but the doorman (or woman) will take one look at you, see an utter lack of rubber, leather, corsetry, or uniforms, and tell you to turn right around and go home.

It's tough to know exactly what a venue expects when they have a dress code in mind; if you have any doubts about whether your fetish outfit will pass muster, try to contact and ask the promoters, look online for pictures from past events, or better yet, talk to people who've been to a similar event or chat with people who work in fetish-wear stores or places that have information about the fetish event (like leather boutiques). Either way, you absolutely must wear fetish attire to attend a fetish event.

Folsom Street Fair, Dore Alley Fair, Slick Fetish Ball, Exotic Erotic, DomDominion (San Francisco); The Black and Blue Ball (New York); German Fetish Ball (Germany); and Skin Two Rubber Ball (UK) are at the time of this writing the largest fetish events in the world, and can be a great (if in some cases expensive) way to experience a large-scale fetish event. Most major cities have big fetish events yearly, and all major cities have a fetish club or monthly night at a local bar where fetish people can dress up and congregate. If you're traveling, it can be a fabulous way to see and experience a new city and meet like-minded kinky people. Do online research before you go to any fetish event to see if there's a message board, or check your local craigslist for people looking for partners or dates to go with.

Keep in mind that there is a spectrum of activity to be found at any given fetish party; some people will only be interested in showing up, looking good, and mingling. Is it just a nightclub, or is it a play space? Find out. Can regular people (like us) use the equipment? Some gatherings might have a strict no-alcohol or drug policy in addition to their dress codes. Still other events and parties might have S/M activities, performances, sex play spaces, or may even have some but not all of these things, or may have to adhere to local laws which might allow S/M activity but no public nudity. When in doubt, ask; many events and parties will have a list of rules to follow. Fetish events are always very sexy in mood and tone, though not all will be okay with nudity, sexual contact, or sometimes even cruising. Still others may have all-out orgy rooms, but with strict "ask before you touch" rules. Violate the rules, and you may be ejected from the party, humiliated (not in a hot fetish way), or barred from attending future events.

Keep your expectations in check when attending one of these events. Just because the revelers will be sophisticated in dress doesn't mean you won't encounter inappropriate drunks, couples fighting, and possibly sexual displays you may not want to see. At the very least, bring the expectation to see some really interesting outfits, and maybe meet a few new people, but not always—even the most perfectly cos-tumed pro domme with the finest looking slaves can go to a fetish party and have no one talk to her all night, and leave feeling abraded by attitude. There is an air of exclusivity at all fetish events, and sometimes it's like being in the cool club and you can relax and feel sexy; other times it's like feeling forever on the outside. More often than not, fetish events are what my good friend calls a "bring-your-own-party kind of party."

Chapter 6
Human Animals

In his early forties, with short graying hair, sharp blue eyes, chiseled laugh lines, and Calvin Klein eyeglass frames, Scott doesn't look like the kind of man who'd love pony play. Indeed, when he teaches to the multitude of students that flow through his UC class every semester, students are known to swoon and try a little harder for a bit of extra attention with their homework, and bloom in praise under his handsome, rugged guidance.

Scott grew up on a farm, far from the city he now teaches in and calls home. But the smell of a tack shop does something to him, something erotic. It reminds him of his early explorations with girls in the stables, times spent in deep connection with his horses, and the ritual of care and grooming. Scott's discovery of the joys of anal play with his female lovers led to fun and games with a horse-hair butt plug bought in a moment of whimsy by a girlfriend who knew Scott loved all things horse-related. But once the plug was in, Scott felt like a pony. And with a loving, nurturing partner, Scott entered the world of ponyboys and their riders. No one knows to look at him, as he looks just like anyone else, but his spirit and libido soar when his girlfriends make him into a sexual pony, one who exists only for their riding pleasure.

Scott is a real person. But Scott's entry into human animal play is only one way in which people come to enjoy this sophisticated style of role-play. Ponies, dogs, cats, farm animals—there are thousands of fetishists worldwide who relish their lives as erotic animals. When in their animal roles, they are groomed, trained to perform, receive behavioral punishment, are "bred" with other animals, outfitted with costumes and gear, and much more.

People who role-play as animals have a variety of reasons for doing so, ranging from a desire to be nurtured, controlled, appreciated, and totally taken care of, all the way to willing explorations of their own psychologies, sexual desires to be "used," to do something taboo, or to become something completely different than who they are in their everyday lives. Across the board, while human animal play goes deep into territory some people might find uncomfortable—sex with animals—human animal play is far from bestiality, or a desire to have sex with actual animals. Just because a couple enjoys pretend sex in the roles of two dogs in heat does not mean they want to have sex with real dogs. Human animal play is not a repressed desire or an expression of a desire to engage in bestiality. People who want to have sex with animals do so; people who want to play as human animals enjoy consensual adult animal role-play scenarios. Big difference.

In animal training, a person is transformed into an animal version of themselves and trained, punished, displayed, kept, or sexually played with as a beast. Overall, it's an advanced form of role-play that may or may not be taken very seriously by the people involved; it can be a silly lark, as in "Bark for me, baby!" Or it can be a deeply spiritual and psychological transformation experience, emotional and grounding. Likely, it's a little of both, or the experience of the players falls somewhere within a spectrum of fun and personal identity. That's not to say that being your sweetie's pussycat or puppy isn't sexy, but it's important to know that human animal play doesn't always involve sex.

There are multitudes of ways to enjoy animal role-play scenarios, from the simple to the advanced. Maybe your fun and games are best when it's just you and your lover under the covers, talking about what you'd do if she needed to be bred with a waiting stable of horny stallions, having sex in your regular ways but with a little fantasy thrown in for extra heat. Or, perhaps your biggest fantasy is to be completely changed from a human into your horse persona, complete with bridle, hooves, grooming, stabling and pony training, ending up in an actual barn full of other human ponies—because such things do exist. Regardless, there is no right or wrong way to enjoy human animal play—only the limits of your imagination.

Role-play with human beasts may or may not be part of a BDSM experience for you; some people will find it heightens the eroticism and strengthens the roles between dominant and submissive, and animal training and care fall neatly into an S/M context. For many, this is a power-play scenario, plain and simple: owner and owned. Conversely, you don't need to be into anything even remotely related to tops and bottoms, whips and chains, or anything else associated with BDSM. For you, animal play is naughty playtime, or an extension of your intimacy and caring for each other.

While most human animals transform into beasts while staying the same gender as their human version, animal play is also an excellent stage for gender transformation as well. In fact, some female humans might identify more strongly or feel hornier as boy dogs, ready to hump their master's leg at the first available moment. Gender animal transformations might unhinge the sexual or psychological aspects needed for a really satisfying experience as the animal, and it may also be a very powerful feeling, a deep desire finally met.

What's great about being a human animal:
- You can be owned
- Someone takes care of your physical needs
- You are treasured, special
- You might be allowed into places humans might not be able to go
- Can be bred with other animals
- Your owner can make you to do things even if you don't want to
- Your life is up to someone else; no decisions to make
- Sex is reduced to animal urges
- It feels good (and smells good) to wear the gear
- If you are bad, you are punished: a very simple exchange
- Being washed by someone else feels amazing
- It feels good to please your keeper/owner
- Lack of human speech allows you to communicate in different ways

- You can explore your self-image in interesting ways
- Your relationship is cemented with a new kind of trust, intimacy and understanding
- You feel beautiful as an animal (being a dirty nasty stinky animal is nice, too)
- You feel powerful

What's great about owning or keeping a human animal:
- Your love for the animal and person is combined
- You're in total control of your lover's welfare, happiness, and sexual satisfaction
- You can be as naughty as you want with their animal self; puppy can't/won't tell anyone you put peanut butter on your pussy and made him lick it off
- Your love and intimacy can be expressed in concrete ways: praise, training, rewards, grooming
- The exchange with your lover is simple, for once: Good gets a reward, bad gets punished
- It's fun; it's a turn-on
- They are completely at your disposal for any whim you might have
- Your pet looks fabulous in their animal gear
- You get a chance to totally "take care" of your lover, which can be especially healing during times of real-life stress
- It cements your BDSM role as top, or it's the perfect vehicle for your overpowerment fantasies
- Paper and slippers delivered on a regular basis

Popular Pets: Ponies and Dogs
While the type, genus, and species of animals and creatures available for this fetish are infinite in number,

like *Animal Farm*, a few rise to the top in popularity and typify the fetish. Horses (ponies), dogs, and pigs occupy the most notorious spots in the fetish bestiary, and by taking a look at how pony and dog fetishes express themselves, you can get an ideas for your own animal scenes and gain understanding into the appeal (and nuts and bolts) of beast fetish play. In any animal scenario, it's good to begin with a clear idea of what you want to do with your scene, what happens in your interactions, and you'll want to test out any outfits, harnesses, or gear beforehand if possible. Human animals might want to spend time alone before the scenario at least once, to practice the walk, gait, actions, sounds of the animal they're going to become, and to get into the physical head space. Being an animal is all about being physical and having a few basic wants and needs. Look in the resources chapter at the end of this book for places to shop, community resources, and ideas for making your own gear.

Pony Play

It stands to reason that sexualized pony play has been around since humans and horses formed their first work relationships; no doubt the concept of riding an animal and euphemisms for sex certainly participated with the rise of the fetish. Most recently (and most popularly), BDSM and fetish ponies in the form of ponygirls and subordinate males made into steeds of varying kinds were seen in art and photography from the 1950s, à la John Willie and Irving Klaw. *Bizarre Magazine* began in the 1950s as an underground extreme fetish publication, influenced a generation of artists, photographers, and fetishists, then disappeared—until the 1980s, when the film *The Perils of Gwendolyne* featured a segment with sexy topless ponygirls doing horsie labor. Next, Anne Rice's *The Claiming of Sleeping Beauty* series of novels about an all-girl horse-training center cracked a signal whip for thousands of horny readers. A pop-culture momentum was reached in the 1990s when Bettie Page and fetish imagery from the era became trendy, and renowned book publisher Taschen re-released the works of Willie and four volumes containing the entire collection of *Bizarre Magazine*, and a flood of sexy human pony imagery hit the markets.

In most pony play one of the participants becomes a horse, while another participant is a fellow horse, a trainer, a passerby, or any other role that sees the pony and recognizes it as such. But while the thrill of simply being equine might be enough for some people, many have a particular type of horse or pony that they like to be, and see their time as a pony, or training one, served in very specific ways.

Cart ponies, like the ones in John Willie's Gwendoline cartoons, are ponies whose main purpose is to be hitched to a cart and pull riders or loads to and fro. This is done with elaborate settings and gear (custom-made human pony carts and rigging, blinders, dress such as plumes and ribbons), or with basic, improvised equipment such as handmade harnesses and modified carriages. At pony fetish events, cart ponies might compete in cart-pulling contests and races. Working horses are the more rugged and muscular version of carthorses, and are expected to haul heavy loads and perform tasks that test the working horse. In some competitions, workhorses are blindfolded and made to haul heavy loads through an obstacle course while interpreting their trainers' signals (without visual cues). They usually have very plain and practical gear and are less about show and more about function and athletic ability.

"Riding ponies" are exactly what the name says: human ponies ridden by their human counterparts. Riding can range from human saddles designed to support the weight of another human on the pony's upright back, to barebacking, where the pony remains on all fours and is ridden about erotically, to everything in between. Generally, riding in outdoor settings and for extended periods is done in an upright fashion as it's easier on the pony's back, and some even see the hands-and-knees approach as unsophisticated. It's just as easy, however, to spring for a pair of kneepads for your pony at Home Depot, so it's up to what you both think will be sexy, practical, and fun. Make sure before you even begin that you're aware of all your pony's potential and actual health problems; back problems or knee injuries will need to be considered before the riding begins.

Show ponies are especially beautiful animals that are groomed in detail, as this may be at the heart of the fetish, and then are shown, exhibited or even entered into contests with other show ponies at pony fetish events. Dressage ponies qualify as show animals, and while simple show ponies must learn dressage gaits, dressage ponies must be able to perform these gaits with grace and style both alone and with a rider.

There are many other types of ponies on the range: While one can be a colt, filly, stallion, or mare, one might also be a gelding or a wild pony. Each of these types of ponies will have to be treated as such—your gelding may have to be examined repeatedly; the wild pony might need to be caught and broken; your stallion may need relief; the mare might need to be bred. Further categories include humiliation ponies (for elaborate ridicule experiences), pleasure ponies (used for sexual gratification), rubber ponies (with special rubber gear or costuming), sissy ponies (typically male humans made into female ponies), and more. It's quite common for a pony persona or style of pony play to overlap into several categories.

You don't need pony gear or special outfits to enjoy horse play, though some people really relish the trappings and costuming. You can just as easily ride your mare in her French maid's outfit, nude or in a custom-made leather-and-satin show-pony costume. Pony saddles, bit gags, bridles, blinders, tails made from actual horse hair (as in a horse-hair butt plug or harness), foot coverings to create hooves, manes—it can all be a very costly habit, but dedicated pony fetishists wouldn't have it any other way. Not everyone has this kind of money to spend on even their most meaningful fetish, so there are plenty of online pony forums with tips and designs for inexpensive DIY pony gear. Think about it—you may not be able to afford pony hooves, but a pair of sexy cloppy-sounding shoes can be the pony shoes that make her transformation complete. Similarly, you can easily improvise a necktie into a bridle, or even simply designate a special satin pillowcase as the one ritual item used only when she's a pony—and you putting it on her as her saddle blanket signifies the instant of her transformation from human to animal.

Ponies need training, exercise, grooming, and good nutrition. Sugar cubes are cute, but carrots are much better for them—and while it seems like I'm being silly, it might just add to your fantasy to create a trough or feed-bag to strap on your pony, filled with delicious honey-sweetened oats (or something to suitably mimic horse chow, like breakfast cereal). Needless to say, tack shops and hardware stores will provide a highly erotic shopping experience for both of you, and there you'll be able to find a variety of items to be used and modified for use in grooming, riding, harnessing, and feeding.

When your pony isn't in service on all fours in its kneepads, she or he will be an upright pony. Don't jump right in and "bit" the mouth of your pony, especially if you're new players. You'll want your first sessions to go slow (and all training should move slowly, for that matter) and you'll want to be able to communicate with your new pony until you both have an understanding and good communication. Ponies on two legs typically have their hands bound behind the back, and must practice balance, carrying passengers or loads, and a variety of gaits (fast, slow and varied). The basic pony step has the knee rising to hip level; show gaits will bring the knees higher. Gaits to train for include walking, moving backward, fancy high-step dressage and show gaits, trots and gallops. Two ponies harnessed together, as in pairs of cart ponies, will need to train and practice walking together, especially in a circle where movements will need to be coordinated between ponies.

Dogs and Pups

While on the surface, dog play may not be as elaborate as pony play, don't be fooled by the lack of saddles and bridles when it comes to the variety of pups to be found at the pound, what they might like to do on any given day and how much gear you can have when you own a human dog. Equipment can include regular dog accessories found at any pet store, such as food and water dishes, water bottles, chains, leashes, collars, choke collars, tags, leashes, tie-downs, toys, blankets, beds, travel crate (or claustrophobia crate), mock kennels, and grooming/cleaning implements.

And don't forget how much fun you can have with a pup when you add BDSM toys to the mix: Dress your doggie up in tails (butt plug–style if you like), paws, ears, harness, knee pads, and even fur, rubber, or full costumes. Mind you, it doesn't take expensive S/M toys to make this happen, but it certainly can add to the physicality of becoming a dog. Good dog, bad puppy—what kind is yours?

Show dogs might just be the princes and princesses of this world, and might be prissy, proud, or even arrogant. Proper training means that posture and intense focus on their master's commands is essential. Learning to follow signals and respond properly is of the utmost importance. Watch dog show competitions, or even the dog-show spoof *Best in Show* for pointers; note how the dogs watch their trainers and carry themselves. These dogs are typically quiet and dignified.

Puppies might be someone who is new to dog play, or it might be the style of dog play they prefer. Puppies behave much like their real-life counterparts: playful, sloppy, spunky, impetuous, willing to try anything and in dire need of training.

Working dogs and guard dogs are focused, strong, and fierce. They can be guide dogs, hearing assistants, or competitive work dogs, such as a collie that herds sheep, runs obstacle courses, or follows very specific commands from its master. Junkyard dogs and other guard dogs tend to be more dangerous and less submissive, so these fierce work animals are great in animal-dominant fantasies.

Stray and wolf dogs are more unpredictable than the rest, and scenarios can range from wild-animal scenes to "breaking" and mastering the wild beast. These dogs have no masters, but may be spotted at fetish parties and events by wearing a chain, collar, or lock with a key in it, signifying availability. Wolves are wild at heart at all times, and may never be trained, but their affection and loyalty can be intense. At its essence, mastering a wolf dog is a power-exchange scenario.

People who interact with dogs might be their owners, a friend of the owner (the dog-sitting scenario), a dog trainer, groomer, or just the BDSM top, no titles necessary. Generally, dogs might need to learn paper-training and basic commands; they need to be fed, exercised, groomed and washed, played with, disciplined if needed, and watched carefully so they don't disobey or get into mischief. There aren't many organizations that have regular human-dog events, but this fetish is welcome at almost every fetish event and dungeon worldwide.

A Bestiary: Other Animals and Fantasy Creatures

Just as the whole world's a zoo, so can be the bedroom. Pigs, cats, tigers, bears, snakes, and even space creatures, mythical beasts, and animals with special powers are all fairly popular fetishes. They might like to pretend to be a fantasy creature and fight or have animal sex, or may enjoy playing the helpless human, or having you play the helpless human. Each creature fetish optimizes the fantasy of occupying the physicality of each creature, and therein lies the attraction.

Plushies and Furries

Plushies and furries have a population large enough to hold their own conventions, and occupy a sizeable part of cyberspace real estate. Plushie is the term typically used to refer to someone who likes to have sex or erotic interaction with stuffed animals, though some in the fetish community will argue that this term is incorrectly used, claiming plushie is actually the name given to the stuffed creature itself and plushophile is the proper name of the human interacting with the stuffed plushie. The stuffed animal can range in size from small to human-sized, can be a puppet, and is usually made in the form of some kind of animal—bears, tigers, and bunnies being the most popular.

Plushophiles might like to collect plushies, sleep, cuddle or have sex with them, or have some sort of intimate relationship with their plushie—much like as a child would, though with the adult reasoning to understand the differences. Plushophiles might like to cuddle the stuffed creature while masturbating, or rub against the fur of the plushie until achieving orgasm. Some modify their plushies to form a space for penetration by opening a seam or adding a masturbation sleeve, or they add a dildo, vibrator, or penetration attachment. Some plushophiles have such strong eroticism for their plushies that they can make themselves come just by looking at one. Other fetishes combine with plush sex and involving partners is even more fun. Rubbing a plushie against your lover's body is fun, as is sandwiching yourself, your lover, or the plushie between you.

Some—but not all—plushophiles are furries, and the two fetish subcultures are often confused by a pop culture that likes to make fun of the culture without taking a minute to get their facts straight. The term "furry" might also describe someone who is interested in animals, furry characters, fursuits, plushies or anthropomorphic characters. Even though there's an element of youth in many aspects of plushophilia and furry fandom, these people have no interest in sex with animals or children; plushophiles and furries are into adult furry sex and sex with their stuffed animals, thank you very much. As I explained at the beginning of this book, these fetishes are not substitutes for adult relationships and intimacy; most often they're an enjoyable adjunct to the healthy adult relationships already in place.

Furries dress in fursuits or "zoots" (the oversize costumes one might see in an amusement park or at sports events on team mascots) and are typically based on fictional characters that have both human and animal attributes. Since a person wearing a fursuit can look and feel a lot like a large living plushie, these costumes are usually quite popular among plushophiles. Furries often make their own fursuits, or they purchase store-bought or custom-made versions of what they like. Other names for a fursuit can include "animal costume," "animal mascot," "zoot," and "zoot suit." One who wears a fursuit might be called a zootaphile, costumer, mascot, or fursuitophile. Some of these costumes have easily accessible genital openings. Some fetishists like to hump or have sex with people wearing these costumes, others like to wear the costumes, and many playact as the actual animals or animal characters in a sexual context.

Furry fans might consider themselves different than the suited furries, though it's common for the subcultures to overlap. A furry fan is someone who enjoys, collects, or fetishizes characters and artwork pertaining to and depicting anthropomorphic creatures, such as talking animals or sexy Japanese fox girls—it's someone who fetishizes part or all of these interests. Furry fandom has ties in sci-fi, comic, cosplay, superhero, and fantasy subcultures, but the principal fetish is for humanized animals, typically sexy ones. Pictures, artwork, live action role-play (LARPing), and general interest in furry creatures fuel the fetish.

Good Dog
Thomas Roche

She rattled the leash as she led him out of his cage into the living room. The feel of the collar around his neck was tight, the leash going taut as he struggled to keep up with her—crawling on all fours, the carpet abrading his knees and palms.

She was nude except for her boots—high-heeled, black patent affairs that came almost to her knees. Down low as he was, he could smell her sex, ripe and musky and close.

She stopped in front of the arm chair, turned to regard him. "Stop!" she said firmly. "Sit. Stay."

He obeyed, sitting on his haunches and looking up at her expectantly. He made a soft "ruff" sound. She bent forward and caressed his hair.

"We're not going for a W-A-L-K right now, Rex. You'll just have to hold it."

Rex uttered a plaintive whine, and she snapped her fingers. "Stop!" she said firmly.

He grew silent, staring up at her desperately. He had been in his cage for three hours, had eaten his dinner from a bowl without the benefit of hands, and licked his mouth clean while she watched him. He had lapped water from another bowl, his chin dripping. Now that water filled his bladder, straining it even as his cock hardened with each stern command she gave him.

"You're a very good doggy, so far," she said. "You've responded very well to your training. But do you know what a good doggy does for his Mistress?"

He cocked his head, looking blankly up at her; he knew better than to respond verbally or even to show any understanding. When he'd done that to her questions before, he'd gotten the newspaper across his ass. It still stung.

She smiled and sat down in the armchair, luxuriously sinking into the red velvet fabric. Her legs spread, she cocked her knees over the arms of the chair, revealing her trimmed pussy. She nudged her body forward until her ass was at the edge of the chair, her vulva lips spread and her cunt glistening luscious in the candlelight.

Then she began to wrap the leash around her hand, slowly pulling him toward her.

She drew his face between her spread legs, cinching the leash tight and pressing his mouth to her cunt. Obediently, he began to lick. She moaned softly. When he began to gently suckle her clit, she snapped: "Bad dog! Lick!" and he returned to licking. Dogs did not suck. They could only lick. He licked obediently, rhythmically, as deeply as he could, from her moist entrance to her swollen clit. His bladder throbbed as his cock grew still harder. He licked fervently, and when he went too quick he got a gentle swat across the shoulder. Dogs had to be trained not to hurry. She moaned louder as he licked her more fully, drooling everywhere, servicing her with a canine whimper.

"Good dog," she cooed as her hips began to grind against him, pressing her sex more firmly against his face. "Goooood doggy..."

She was intensely aroused to begin with, so within minutes he had found her rhythm and was swiftly bringing her toward orgasm as his cock pulsed in agony. His bladder full, all he could think of was servicing his Mistress so she would take him for that precious W-A-L-K, allowing him to relieve himself.

She snuggled herself down further on the chair, tightening her grip on the leash. "Don't stop," she said breathlessly. "Don't stop, little doggy...oh!"

Then she came, and he lapped at her enthusiastically as he listened to the cries of her orgasm. Her back arched and she squirmed, her thighs coming together around his face as she pumped her hips. He rode her obediently, taking her to her peak and then feeling her relax under him.

When she was finished, she pushed him back, away from her sex. His mouth dripped her juices. She leaned back in the chair and smiled at him.

"Ready to go for that W-A-L-K now?" she asked.

He knew better than to respond directly. Instead he yipped and reared back on his haunches. But he knew there was no way he could relieve himself with his cock as hard as this. With a smile, she seized a rubber glove from the chair-side table and, deftly negotiating her grip on the leash with her left hand, snapped the glove onto her right.

"Roll over," she said firmly.

He did, his legs in the air, his cock standing straight as she came out of the chair and crouched over him. Her rubber-sheathed hand wrapped around his cock, and he yowled, almost forgetting himself with a moan as she stroked him once, twice, three times very, verrrrry slowly — then began pumping him faster as he approached his release, his bladder pressing painfully the whole time.

When he came, he almost called out from the pain of his

pleasure forcing its way past his swollen bladder. But he remembered himself at the last minute — and barked.

He barked and howled and rolled back and forth on his back as he shot his come onto his hairy belly. Crouching, she smiled and finished him off.

"Good boy," she sighed. "Good doggy. Come on. Time for that W-A-L-K."

He obediently got back onto all fours, not even caring that as he did, he dripped cum all over his carpet. His cock still hurt from the pressure in his full bladder. She unraveled the leash and began to lead him through the house.

As she led him toward the front door, he felt a sudden wave of fear and shame, and responded with a plaintive whine. Even spent as it was, he felt his cock stir with the fear that she would make him pee in the front yard.

She chuckled, as if reading her pet's mind. She took a right turn at the kitchen and led him toward the back door.

"Don't worry," she sighed. "I don't think the world's ready for your brand of canine."

As she led him into the chill of the back yard, toward the bushes, she laughed again.

"Besides," she said as he lifted his leg next to the foot of the azalea tree. "I didn't bring any bags."

His canine face turning red, he let himself go, a hot stream into the thick underbrush through the tightened channel of his painfully softening cock. His Mistress watched as he went, her face bearing a luxurious expression of abject pleasure and pride.

"Good dog," she sighed as he went. "Gooood dog."

Chapter 7
Cross-Dressing and Sissies

For many outsiders, the wild and wooly (or rubbery, if you will) world of fetishes seems like the land of clichés, and that may be true to a certain extent. Fetishes inflate stereotypes, specifics, and fascinations to far-flung reaches. But in the area of fetish reserved for those who wear clothing that belongs to the other gender, clichés become very revealing. Take for instance the saying, "It's a man's world." Women have worked very hard over the past, oh, 100 years or so to turn that phrase upside down—but in the world of cross-dressing fetish and sissy-boys, it's a woman's world indeed. Or a man's world, depending on how you look at it.

Ever since he was a young boy, Mike had a fascination

for women's private undergarments. He found the strange fabrics compelling, alluring, mysterious, exciting. Later, as a teenage boy, he dated girls his age and withheld information about his attraction to their undergarments—namely, that he liked to wear them when no one was around, and it turned him on like nothing he could imagine.

Mike got lucky and dated a sexually open-minded woman who discovered his fascination for women's underwear and indulged him. One evening she made him up in drag, and they went out to a fetish party, paying special attention to his undergarments. It was daring and scary, but for Mike it was an awakening. He'd always felt like he had a horrible secret that made him feel like a freak, but the look and feel of high heels, the softness of satin panties on his genitals, the constriction of nylons, and the transformation afforded by a wig and lipstick sent him over the edge into heaven. He felt sexy, okay to be naughty; he even felt like for once he could ask for his sexual fantasies to come true, and it would be okay. Having broken up with his permissive paramour upon this writing, Mike now only dates only women he hopes will want to play with him, panties and all.

Mike is a cross-dressing fetishist; his fetish is very different than the transgender experience of my friend Angela. She didn't simply fetishize being a man in women's clothing, though her double life often found her keeping company with cross-dressing (CD) fetishists and a spectrum of transgender assimilations. Her secret life had her dressing up and having experiences far from her other life as a married man with a wife and three children, a Harley-Davidson motorcycle, corporate job, and military-officer past. But when Angela put on women's clothing, it was like coming home; she *was* a woman, she wanted to pass, she wanted to just live her life as any other woman might.

It may seem like I'm oversimplifying my point, but this chapter is not meant as a gender discourse; it is not for people who think they might be transgender, born in the wrong body or are interested in transitioning into full-time life as a different gender than the one assigned at birth. It's also not necessarily a drag queen primer, though I say "not necessarily" because cross-dress fetish is enjoyed by primarily straight, gay and bi men—drag is a gay subculture, and while the two may overlap, it's a whole other bag o' makeup. In the context of this fetish, dressing in women's clothing doesn't mean you want to *be* a woman. But maybe it's a turn-on to be treated like one.

If cross-dressing gives you a sexual thrill, read on. If you're in it for kicks; a sexual or psychological release; to feel "bad," "slutty," or "easy"; you enjoy living as your regular gender; you don't care so much about "passing" as the opposite gender. If you see cross-dressing as a punishment and demasculinization as erotic or desirable for whatever reasons, then this chapter is for you and your lovers. However, if all of this overlaps for you, that's just fine—no one ever fits into neat little sexual categories. Maybe you just like panties; perhaps you only feel alive when you're a sissy maid; it could be the finest moment of your life to be forced into women's clothing, fucked with a strap-on, and humiliated and beaten for being a stupid slut. Maybe you just enjoy your feminine "role." Or, it makes you kinda hot to wear your girlfriend's lipstick, nothing more—it's all a spectrum of fetish, and none of it means you're gay, trans, bi, sick, going to "hell," or confused. Actually, you're the opposite of confused; you know what you like and want to do, but likely have a lot of questions. This chapter is primarily geared toward straight males, though if you're neither straight nor male but enjoy fetishizing opposite gender items, you belong here too. If you're in unclear gender or identity territory, relax — and pick up a copy of *My Gender Workbook* by Kate Bornstein.

Cross-dressing isn't typically a politically correct fetish, though if being an empowered female gets you hard, Buffy did have fabulous blowouts (hair) and excellent lip gloss. (Faith was the slutty one; see you *can* have the best of both worlds!) What some people find unnerving about this fetish tends to be the gender stereotypes and exaggerations inherent in the fascination with what makes, say, a woman a woman. Sometimes the way cross-dress fetish manifests itself may not be pretty (ahem), or it might be downright offensive, and it might even make it seem like the man with the fetish has a negative way of perceiving women; not likely, but it's good to ask if you have any of these questions. Just because a man likes to be made into a sissy maid and called a slut doesn't mean he thinks all women are submissive whores (or that they should be). In fact, it might be the opposite. Many men who like becoming submissive females would prefer doing so with female dominants; others may find having a female partner wear a strap-on thrilling; a few might want to go "all the way" and try sex with an actual male partner. A good number of cross-dress fetishists see women as powerful, deserving of respect, mysterious, and all-knowing. This seems like a contradiction, and it is, but it makes perfect sense to the man in the panties. For them, cross-dressing is a manifestation of awe and desire for the opposite sex.

Wearing women's clothing and/or makeup is an entry into a hidden, forbidden world. For men, it is full of secrets — sexy secrets. From makeup tricks to walking in heels, squeezing into tight but soft undergarments to assuming a submissive sexual role (or not; just female) — it's all very far from the world of men, and what it means to be one. A man might see female clothing on his body as making him feel sexy, sexually receptive, okay to let someone else call the shots, or a fun way to play with "lesbian" fantasies, using his giant clit (penis) for fun and games with his new "girlfriend." Taken further, it's permission to let go, not make decisions, to get slapped around or get sexually "used" as a feminine sex object that is so desirable that no one can hold back their lust — they just have to "take" what they want with her. Women live very different sexual lives than men; he might just want to "try on" how the other half lives for a change. It's all about perception, of course, and fantasy, but it's all sex play between adults. And that's how to have fun with it; just play.

Elements of cross-dress fetish, to be enjoyed solo or in combination — use your erotic imagination:

- Women's undergarments: panties, corsets, girdles, nylons and pantyhose, bras, crotchless hose and panties, bloomers, ruffle butt panties
- Other women's or sissy wear: aprons, skirts, dresses, slutwear (tight and revealing spandex, miniskirts, porn star lingerie), cutoff shorts and cutoff tank tops, elegant gowns, maid's outfit, uniforms like cheerleader or nurse, female submissive gear, any female rubber garments, gloves (such as opera length), girlie socks, pinafores, petticoats and frilly hats, sweaters

(cashmere, angora), earrings, ladies' or little girls' jewelry

- Makeup: lipstick, full-face makeup
- Women's shoes: high heels, platforms, "fuck-me" pumps, stripper shoes, go-go boots, thigh-high boots, "hobble" shoes and boots (typically ballerina-style toes, patent leather), Mary Janes, mules (especially feather-trimmed marabou), open-toed sandals, pumps with a slave lock or D-rings on the ankle, stilettos, and spike heels
- Hair: styled or a wig
- Partial or full body shaving
- Outfits/roles: maid, slut, little girl, sissy, princess, schoolgirl, guy in panties, businesswoman, super-heroine, nurse, cheerleader, hooker, waitress
- Scenarios: female service roles, female sexual-service roles, forced feminization, punishment with feminine clothes, getting "caught" in the panty drawer or trying the lipstick, being "discovered" wearing frilly undergarments beneath masculine clothes, being an animal of another gender, role-playing, age-play scenarios, "forced" sex scenarios, dominated and sissified husband, little boy made into little girl, learning what it takes to be a "real woman," discipline schedules, panty punishment
- Further feminization: tucking, prosthetic breasts, cleavage bras, sanitary napkins, strap-on discipline, hair removal

Her Makeup and Hair

If there's one rule when it comes to cross-dressing and hair/makeup choices, there's simply no accounting for taste. Often, fetishes are very specific and nonsensical; it could be that the ugliest, most garish color of lipstick is the one thing that sets your heart racing. Each person will have their own vision or preferences when it comes to hair and makeup, so I won't be giving you advice on looking great for a date, but I will tell you what you need to know to buy makeup discreetly, and how to go all-out for a sexily whorish or diva look, depending on what floats your armada.

Buying makeup is always a quandary, especially in small towns; if you want to do it and retain your privacy, you'll either need to just do it and get it over with at the local drugstore, order online, or shop in a different town. Get an idea together in your head of what you want before you start shopping; is it ruby-red lips and blonde hair? Green eye shadow and braids? Look at pictures of people you'd like to emulate and study the details so you can reproduce them later. Trying the makeup on your skin in person is ideal; that way you can see how it really will look and test for irritation—but since this isn't always possible, always buy non-comodogenic, non-perfumed makeup whenever possible. If you don't know where to start, order or purchase a giant "sampler" kit, usually of low-grade yet inexpensive lipsticks, eye shadows, blushes, bases and nail polish. These provide a lot of variety and let you experiment to find the colors and look you like (try sephora.com).

If you're doing your own makeup, be very patient with yourself. Even if you've been doing it for decades, like me, you can still fuck it up. You will make mistakes, your hand will shake, your eyes will water when you don't want them to; it takes practice. The more you do it, the better you'll get, and that's the only way to learn. Get yourself makeup remover wipes, which allow you to play and remove, and are great for spot-removal. Also, this primer is as basic as it gets—read up on techniques online, take a theatrical makeup class, or buy a great makeup how-to book such as *Making Faces by* Kevyn Aucoin.

You might want, in order of application:
- Liquid base: Industrial-strength bases like Dermablend and Cover Girl's Outlast (and Smoothers) hide stubble well, but there are *many* great drugstore brands. Use a non-oily lotion first or blend lotion with your base so it sinks in. Pat it on with your fingertips and let it settle; be sure to blend around hairline and jawline.
- Concealer, for under-eye circles and blemishes.
- Lipstick (lip liner sucks, but it's great for certain looks where the outlines of the lips are darker than the inside).
- Eyebrows: You can pluck or trim to thin them out, or buy a shaping kit. You may or may not need to draw in more brow; use a light hand to trace your lines on first, and try not to get frustrated if you miss.
- Eye shadow: Lots to experiment with here, but my general advice is to always use a skin-colored shadow all over lids as a base so your other colors go on smoothly. Cream shadows will always cake in the crease of your eyes, but hey, it's a look, too.
- Eye liner: soft pencil, liquid or cream, it's up to you.
- Lashes: You can use mascara and be sure to curl your eyelashes, or you can apply false eyelashes. Curl your lashes with a lash curler, or my favorite, a heated lash

curler (a little battery-operated wand that heats and is easy to use; visit sephora.com). Always put your lashes on last, over the top of your makeup. With false lashes, put glue along the plastic edge and wait a few minutes before applying for the glue to set, then press the outer edge on. With the inside still sticking up, use the edge of something like a pointed chopstick and press the rest into place.

- Makeup may feel strange the first few times you wear it; in fact, it's easy to forget and scratch an itch, ruining your lipstick or eyeliner.

Hair is another realm altogether. My best suggestion is to get a variety of wigs so you can play with color, style, pigtails, braids, and shapes; Halloween and online stores are good for the shy shopper. Be sure to get a hair net to wear under the wig; it'll keep all your stray hairs under control. Wigs are hot and they itch until you get used to them, but they can change the entire look of your face, your makeup, even your outfit and your body shape. I own about ten wigs (and several clip-on hair extensions) of different colors and styles; I highly recommend wigs.

Shoes

The one thing that gets your blood boiling might just be shoes—and shoes alone. Or, they might be the finishing touch on an ensemble that perfectly completes your fetish. Shoes are very personal and intimate; each person will have their own shoe requirements. When you have your dream shoes in mind, you'll likely want to shop in stores that cater to large and men's sizes—and there are plenty of them to be found on the Web (see Chapter 11, "Resources"). It's ideal if you live in a major city with a sizeable drag/trans/cross-dressing population, and have access to their stores; trying on shoes in person is the best way to shop. Shoe sizes vary, and while you might be an 11 in men's regular, you may be a 12 in Foot Worship stiletto sizes, or a 10 1/2 at Dream Dresser. But chances are good that you don't have access to these stores and will need to shop online, both for access and privacy, in which case I urge you to select with care, read return policy information thoroughly, and be prepared to send back and exchange shoes that don't fit at least once in your lifetime—probably more.

The right fit is important, especially when you're talking about extreme fetish shoes, high heels, and hobble boots/shoes. Shoes that are too big might distract from how you feel, or they might add to your playtime illusion in wearing "older sister's" shoes. But if you're going to be wearing heels for any amount of time you'll want them to fit right—your feet are going to hurt no matter what as they adjust to being in shoes you're not used to, and your calf muscles will ache afterward until you build up the right muscles for strutting your stuff.

High heels are remarkable. They are damn sexy; you won't believe how they change the appearance of your feet, ankles, calves, thighs, butt, and even your posture. They create one hell of an erotic transformation. They look sexy, they sound nice on hard floors. Still, they're frustrating to learn to walk in, so be prepared to practice, practice, practice. But for look and feel, there's nothing compared to a hot pair of heels.

Shaving

Invariably, at some point in our lives, we have all shaved some part of our anatomy, and most of us prefer some part of ourselves to be hair-free. The first time was probably tense: a sharp razor, an unsure hand, lather, and a new sensation as blade met skin. But for many of us the result was an unforgettable feeling of silky smooth skin, sensitive to the touch, with all of the bare skin's nerve endings at full attention. This heightened sensitivity and responsiveness is what makes genital shaving so alluring. To learn even more about shaving (and waxing) your genitals, check out the extensive sections in my books *The Ultimate Guide to Cunnilingus* and *The Ultimate Guide to Fellatio*.

The thought of taking a razor and effectively scraping it across our most tender bits, however, is enough to scare many people away from what could be a fun erotic experiment. Or, at least, it's likely to make you feel the same tension and anxiety as the first time you picked up a razor and started shaving any other part of your body. But just like shaving you'd do anywhere else, genital shaving has its own techniques, rules, and tricks for successful de-furring—and some important ways to avoid irritation afterward.

Start out by softening the hair; take a warm bath or shower, using soap and conditioner on your pubic region. When you're through and dry, trim the hair with small scissors, such as mustache trimmers, though I find that electric clippers do a terrific job in a short amount of time. This turns the hair into shavable fuzz, and also gives you an idea of the ground you're about to cover with your razor—you can see where all the hair is.

Get comfortable in front of a mirror. A door- or wall-mounted mirror is ideal, because you can pull up a chair, spread a towel on the seat, and have a clear view. If you don't have a big mirror, you can prop up a small mirror and sit in front of it anywhere that feels comfortable. You can even set it against the back of your chair or against your toilet tank, and sit backwards to face your reflection. When you get settled comfortably, check your lighting: The light should be bright enough to see the individual hairs, and you may need to bring in extra lighting.

Set yourself up with a cup or bowl of warm water, a fresh safety razor, and an extra towel. Use a thick shaving cream or gel. The types designed for sensitive skin (such as Aveeno) are highly recommended. Set the razor in the warm water to heat it up, moisten the area you're about to shave—legs, underarms, scrotum, pubic mound, and anus—and work up a creamy lather with the shaving cream. Apply the lather (which feels pretty good, by the way) and start shaving.

Go slowly and try to shave in the direction the hair grows, if you can tell. Make one short stroke per area your goal—you want to shave with as few repeat strokes as possible. Keep your grip light so the razor can gently follow the contours of rounded areas, and don't press. Rinse your razor in the water after each stroke to keep it clean. With tricky areas, such as your knees or testicles, use your other hand to gently pull and flatten the skin so your razor can glide over it. You'll be surprised to find that hair grows in some unlikely places.

Watch your strokes in the mirror, and if you start to feel like your back is turning into a painful question mark, take a moment to sit up and breathe. Shaving the anal area is tough because it's practically impossible to see, but some people find that it's easier upside down! Try turning around and bending over completely, so you're looking through your legs at your butt in the mirror, and use your free hand to pull your buttocks aside. Squatting over a mirror is also highly recommended. You may think you look silly now, but trust me, it'll feel divine when you're done.

Once you're through, hop back in the shower for a warm (not hot) rinse. Your newly shaved delicates will feel hypersensitive when the water hits, so just gently run your hands over everything to remove the shaving cream. If you can stand it, exfoliate gently with a loofah or exfoliating gloves—exfoliation will be your ongoing helper to avoiding the dreaded shaving itch and ingrown hairs as the hair struggles to return to it rightful place. You can use a little soap if you have some with a low pH, like glycerin, Aveeno, hand-milled, or goat's milk (all unscented). A harsh perfumed soap will irritate your skin, which has just been stripped of all its protective oils, so avoid harsh soaps. If you feel brave, make your final rinse cool water to close your pores.

Pat dry and apply an aftershave treatment to avoid razor burn. When I did research on shaving and waxing, it seemed like everyone had a different way to deal with razor rash—much like when you get a cold and everyone tells you a different home remedy that "really works." Chicken soup for a shaved pussy notwithstanding, many people swear by Neosporin ointment, almond oil, hypo-allergenic lotion, cocoa butter, calendula cream, exfoliation, and aftershaves. These work well for the people who recommended them to me, but I have extremely sensitive skin that erupts in razor burn if I get too close to the razors in a drugstore display case. Zinc oxide creams (sold for diaper rash) work quite well; Desitin and Aveeno (unscented) are also highly recommended. My favorite product on the market that works astoundingly well is something called Tend Skin, though it's a harsh astringent and you will want to use it sparingly. You can get Tend

Skin at sephora.com. Avoid hydrocortisone creams because they thin your skin over time. The first few times you shave, the area will itch like hell when your hair begins to grow back, but this eventually stops. To help with the itch, carry a bottle of light hypo-allergenic lotion with you and apply it as needed, and again, exfoliate whenever you shower.

A lot of the information here may make shaving seem like a difficult process. But many people eroticize the procedure, and some even have their lovers help—or do it for them. Bad "girls" can be punished with a shaving, or sissies might need to be maintained with a regular shave. After your first few shaves, you'll find it gets easier. Eventually, you'll probably be able to simply shave in the shower as part of your routine. You won't believe how bare bits feel beneath your own hands or inside a rubber garment or panties, and it feels incredible during sex—especially oral sex and hand jobs. You'll feel it every time you take a step: smooth skin on panties, boxers, or your jeans. Enjoy the touchable new you—and good luck keeping your hands off yourself!

What Is a Sissy-Boy?

If you've never heard this term in a fetish context before, it's easy to think this is a schoolyard insult, or a derogatory gay slur; actually, this context fits its present use in defining the sissification subculture—and it's bigger than you think. Sissy-boys are submissive males whose role-play is based around a desire to be trained at becoming responsible, disciplined girls or women at the stern and firm hands of a superior; sometimes a pro domme, a partner, or their lover. Cruel schoolmates call effeminate boys sissies; adult sissy fetishists may react to the label in a variety of ways (pride, humiliation, shame, arousal), but taken one way or another it's the term for the submissive feminized male. A significant portion of the sissy culture is devoted to age play, that is, the adult male sissy enjoys playing as a little girl or sometimes a female baby — this is AB play, or adult baby role-play, covered in Chapter 8, "Medical Play and Adult Babies." This section is primarily geared toward grown-up sissy cross-dressers, especially the naughty husband and sissy maid.

Some sissy boys get feminized, others don't. Most get humiliated and punished for infractions and weakness of character, both real and imagined. Sissies are often forced to cross-dress. Regardless, sissies always value the superiority and value of a woman, and seek to become like her through worship, service, and discipline.

What happens to sissies:
- Sissies require constant reminders of their place, which is groveling at your feet.
- They get smacked in the face or on the rump when they misbehave.
- They are "made" to dress up in things like makeup, perfume, frilly undergarments, teen and training bras, knee-high socks and Mary Janes, Catholic schoolgirl uniforms, maid outfits in rubber or satin, party dresses, press-on nails, and high heels.
- You can make sissy put on shows for you: dancing, stripping, singing, or "clit milking."
- Sissy's discipline comes from doing his chores; dress him up and make him do housework.
- Put panties on your sissy and make him scrub the floor or give you a pedicure.

- Teach sissy to do your hair and makeup, and help you get dressed.
- Sissy maids get special uniforms but must adhere to strict behaviors, even while doing housework and chores. You may decide if your sissy gets punished for infractions or good behavior, but be consistent — sissies are impressionable and only understand repeated behavior training. At home, plan a special maid's day where sissy is a maid all day long. You can make sissy wait on you and your girlfriends for an afternoon of tea, or you can lend sissy out to your friends for their entertainment and special training. Read advanced sissy-maid training techniques in *A Charm School for Sissy Maids* and *The Mistress Manual* by Mistress Lorelei.
- Make sissy wash all your dirty panties or polish all your shoes.
- Scold and humiliate him for being such a sissy; point with your finger and make fun of his tiny soft little clit (but it might not stay tiny or soft during the berating).
- Fuss over your sissy; forcibly fix hair, wipe smudges from his face, cruelly adjust his clothing.
- Sissies get spanked. A lot.
- They also get strap-on discipline.
- They get panty punishments of all kinds — read on.

Forced feminization tips for the dominant partner:
- Use many of the above feminine punishment suggestions for your scene, depending on what you negotiate with your submissive will enhance the experience of being forced into womanhood.
- Think about the feminization beforehand and be

sure you assemble gear, clothing, makeup and other accoutrements to create the sappiest, most cliché version of femininity possible, especially if humiliation is an important part of the scene.

- Map your scene in at least four basic parts: establishing your dominance, forcing "her" into her feminine clothes and makeup, a climax that involves transgression and punishment, then a finale where the girly redeems herself through sexual service and rededication to her mistress.
- To set the scene, lay out all the things you'll use, and create suspense by having hidden tools at your disposal that you allude to, such as a special hairbrush for mistake corrections (spanking) or panties for gagging sissy girls who mouth off or cry too much.
- Begin by explaining who you are and her role; maybe you're a headmistress or goddess and she needs to learn to be a real woman — or is a slut needing to be taught a lesson.
- Dress her up and put her makeup on, explaining everything along the way, reminding her that you're introducing her to the mysterious world of women's secrets. You can make it hurt if it pleases you.
- Make her perform a task for you: dancing, a striptease, tea service, laundry.
- If she doesn't fuck it up somehow, stick out a leg and trip her.
- Tell her she has a lot to learn as a woman and you'll have to teach it to her. Then punish in a previously agreed upon manner, such as panty gagging and whipping, or strap-on teaching so she can learn to

service a man (cocksucking and ass-fucking), or crawling on her hands and knees while you ride her.

- Angrily try to fix her hair and makeup afterward.
- Tell her she can make it up to you, explain exactly how, and have her do so immediately — never withhold forgiveness after a punishment unless you've agreed on this beforehand, as this can be a particularly cruel emotional punishment.
- She has earned the right, through pain and humiliation, to perform an intimate task for you. Have her make it up to you by servicing you sexually — instruct her in the oral ways of "lesbians" so she can learn to please you correctly. Or, have her give you a massage or bathe you.
- Tell her what a beautiful girl she is and that you are pleased. If you so choose, you may tenderly remove her makeup and dry her off after she bathes. You may also allow her sexual release, if it hasn't already been part of the scenario. You can also continue the scene until you decide she may have an orgasm — as long as you like.

Panties and Panty Punishment

Panties are irresistible: They're soft, intimate, and when still warm or smell, it can put your panty-boy fetishist into overdrive. Not all panty boys are sissies, but panty punishment is a universal language. Panty boys might be sniffers, thieves, panty sluts wanting to be forced into sex while wearing panties, need to be gagged or blinded with panties while unspeakable sexual things happen, or he may have to put on special shows in his, or your, panties.

Panty punishments come in a variety of flavors; never forget that panties are how you show him who's in charge. You can panty him and force him to wear his panties under his work clothes all day so he thinks of you every time he shifts or needs to use the bathroom stall to pee instead of the urinal. Similarly, you can panty him and make him do anything your heart desires. You may have a special pair of punishment panties to make him wear when he's been bad, and they may signify when he's going to get spanked, whipped, or receive strap-on discipline. Use your hand for panty-punishment spankings only if you absolutely must—how *hateful* to break a nail on panty-boy's behind. Use a paddle or "womanly" tool, such as a kitchen implement like a wooden spoon.

The panties may be your poor (wo)man's chastity device, and he should not be allowed to touch or pleasure himself as long as he's pantied—until you say so. His panties might have companion accessories such as a leash, collar, and lipstick. The frillier the better? Why not! Never let him take his panties off (or put them on) without your approval. You may have to inspect his panties frequently for mysterious stains and follow proper behavior training for "accidents." Oral service in panties is also a fine punishment choice, especially if he's not allowed to touch himself during his service.

Girls' School
Thomas Roche

"You've been reported to my office," she said breathily into his ear, "for moral transgressions. Your dorm-mates say that you've been *masturbating* in your bunk bed at night."

Her hand traveled down the front of his body, nearing his quickly stiffening cock. He gulped.

"Is this true, Charlie?"

There were no costumes, no setting, no setup, no warning—they were both nude, in bed, ready for sleep except for the powerful erotic hunger Justine had just conjured between them. With a few firmly spoken words, she'd rendered him as a schoolgirl as surely as if she'd dressed him up in a uniform-regulation plaid skirt. And Charles just *went* with it, because they'd played a close enough game more than enough times that the turn-on, while undeniably exotic, was also soothingly familiar.

"N–no, Headmistress. I don't know what you're talking about. I'd never do something like that."

He liked that touch, augmenting the fantasy a little— she was the Headmistress of a strict girls' school, where "moral crimes" were forbidden. When her hand wrapped around his naked cock, he gave a little moan.

"Then why is your clit becoming hard just talking about it?" she growled, gripping hard—hard enough to feel good, and then hard enough to hurt, as she pressed her naked body against his. "Clearly you have needs that you're tempted by. Have you been eating spicy food?"

"No, Headmistress."

"More than your ration of meat?"

"No, Headmistress."

"Looking at the other girls when they pass by in their gym clothes?"

He squirmed against her grasp on his cock, struggling not to grind his hips against her stroke.

"N—no, Headmistress."

She laughed. "That's ridiculous. I've seen you looking, Charlie. I've seen you watching them as they pass. I've seen you lusting after their tight little bodies. You think a girl your own age can see to this?" She indicated his cock with a squeeze. "You think a high school girl could satisfy it better than your Headmistress?"

"No, Headmistress," he said, his voice strained.

She kissed him, hard, reaching down to grip his balls, squeezing enough to make him writhe. When their lips parted she laughed, and began to stroke his cock slowly up and down, jerking him off.

"You're a fool to even look at other girls your own age. Let me show you what a real woman can do, Charlie. And then we'll see if you need to touch your little clit at night." She stroked harder, kissing him, pressing her breasts tight against his chest, picking up the pace as his back arched and he whimpered with his approaching orgasm.

She gave a cruel laugh and added: "From now on, Charlie, when you feel that need, no matter what time of day or night, I want you in my quarters. I want you to show up at my door and tell me 'Headmistress, my clit is hard.' Do you understand?"

He responded with a moan.

She squeezed his cock harder, stroked violently, pumping it up and down. "I said, do you understand?" she snapped.

He threw his head back and moaned, "Yes, yes, I understand" —just before he came, uttering a bestial groan and pumping his hips forward into her grasp. She finished him off with a neat series of strokes, laughing as his come shot and pulsed and then drizzled out.

"There," she sighed, cuddling against him. "Could one of those tarts in gym shorts do that for you? Could your own hand do that as good as I do?"

"No, Headmistress."

"Then what are you going to do when your little clitty gets hard, Charlie-girl? Day or night?"

"Come to you, Headmistress."

"Good, Charles. No more touching yourself."

"Yes, Headmistress."

"From now on, *I'm* the only one who touches you."

He sighed and pulled her close.

Chapter 8
Medical Play and Adult Babies

At first glance, the name of this chapter might be confusing for at least one reason: How do these two seemingly incongruent fetishes go together? It's easy to see why I chose to put them in the same chapter when you boil down their basic elements and discover that these extreme power-exchange, role-based caretaking fetishes have a lot in common, even though they differ in some pretty important ways.

While a good many practicing medical fetishists and infantilists may not want these fetishes to mix, they have a lot in common. Adult babies like to be taken care of, to be pampered, to give up total control to an all-knowing mommy or daddy who holds their happiness (and punishment) in their hands. Adult babies are swaddled in diapers; are fussed over in a nearly medical, though very maternal, way with feedings and temperature-takings; and their caretakers are sometimes menacing and cruel. Mommy or daddy can enjoy the complete power and control they have over their charge and exact very adult penance, punishment, and pleasure from their "baby." Humiliation might be an essential component in the fetish. They can also nurture their tot and dress baby up for different occasions. Gender roles and their stereotypes in this context are often extremely important. Sometimes the adult role in the scenario is a nurse, doctor, or wet-nurse.

Medical play involves naughty nurses, sexy doctors, and their patients—another power-over scenario that is clearly defined. Typically, medical role-play is in an adult-role context, though not always, and a good number of fantasies may involve age regression on the part of the patient. Patients need to be fussed over with medial accuracy; must strip down and don gowns and bandages, or be nude; and are subjected to examinations and physical ordeals. Nurses and doctors can be doing it for the patient's "own good," be nurturing in their care, or frighteningly sinister. Humiliation might be the desired state of the patient; gender roles are often very important in creating a satisfying encounter.

These two fetishes are "caretaking" fetishes because they typify the sexual scenario in which one role is the caretaker or guardian of well-being of the submissive (who has given up total control), and there is a strong element of captivity and vulnerability as well. Caretaking is actually a huge component in many scene or role-based fetishes, such as animal play and other fetishes that involve bondage, physical restraint, and clear power-exchange dynamics. But here, we see everyday human roles pulled from somewhat real-life situations and fetishized to some pretty amazing, sexy, and intense extremes.

Medical Fetish

Simply put, medical fetishes involve some sort of medical captivity, examination, and power exchange between the patient and medical "professional." Uniforms, medical instruments, bandages, examinations, and atmosphere are important elements, but specifics will differ from person to person. Sometimes the patient is rendered physically helpless from a medical condition; perhaps they're being examined and given some kind of physical (sexual and/or painful) "medicine." The most common manifestation is of course the "naughty nurse" or "sexy doctor" seduction fantasy, though medical fetishists are usually in it for more than an *ER* role-play scene; some medical fetishists may orgasm simply from the feel (or sight or sound) of cold stainless-steel medical instruments. Some fantasies might involve an evil doctor and science experiments, enema play, catheterization, dental gags, medical sounds (stainless-steel rods), gynecological tools and exams, daily rituals of hospital life, surgery fantasies, bandages and casts, wheelchair and orthopedic confinement, and sexual abuse by various types of medical staff.

Predicaments

It's possible that you or you lover have an interest in medical fetish but don't know where to get started. Or maybe one of you has a fetish and would like a few ideas to show to your lover so you can skip happily into the hospital together for fun and games. The best advice for med beginners is to start slow. Begin with outfits—agree on your roles and get together a nurse's or doctor's uniform and decide what your patient will wear (see resources chapter for shopping recommendations).

- Novice doctors will want: a white coat, nametag, stethoscope, pens, gloves (latex or nitrile), a clipboard, and slacks. Your outfit may also depend on what kind of doctor you are.
- Surgeons wear scrubs: usually green drawstring pants, matching smock (top), gloves (latex or nitrile), paper booties over shoes, paper shower-style cap, mask, and possibly goggles or glasses.
- Mad doctors might want: any or all of the above, with crazy hair, aviator's goggles, and rubber apron.
- Nurses wear: crisp white uniforms (usually a whole dress), nurse's cap with a red cross, stethoscope, pens, clipboard, latex or nitrile gloves, white stockings or tights, white shoes. Of course, modern nurses seldom dress like this anymore, so if realism is your thing, look at the wide variety of unisex smocks available that come in many colors and patterns. Rubber may be an essential element to the fetish, and rubber nurse uniforms are widely available; for more info, read Chapter 5, "Fetish Dressing."
- Patients might be: in regular clothes that need to come off, either voluntarily or removed with medical scissors (clothes you don't care about); nude; or wearing bandages, leg or arm braces, paper gowns, or revealing pajamas.

What happens in a medical scene:

- Patient is subjected to examination, which may include temperature taking-(rectal or otherwise, can use fingers, penis, butt plug), cavity exams, etc.
- Patient makes appointment with doctor or nurse (a great way to call and set up your scene for later) with an ailment that needs treatment—or is imaginary.
- Doctor subjects patient to humiliating or painful exam, or sexually compromising treatment.
- Medical bathing or sponge baths
- Bandaging or application of orthopedics, or casts (or sex in these items)
- Supervised urination or defecation
- Forced sex
- Body shaving (see shaving section in the cross-dressing chapter)
- Mock surgery (with mask for patient), mock cutting, and fake blood
- Extreme bandaging, or mummification, especially if bandages leave patient sexually available and unable to move
- Horrifying experiments
- Treatment and medicines for ailments may involve orgasm therapy, penis or pussy milking, anal therapy, sexual service to the doctor or nurse, S/M (whipping, spanking, caning, etc.), sensory deprivation, and orifice or body-part stretching. Medical personnel can also administer (fake) pills and therapeutic drinks. Advanced treatments include anal or bladder enemas, catheterization, piercing, cupping, fire, speculum exams, body-part inflation with saline injections, and urethral sounds.

Tools of the trade vary, of course, depending on what scenario you find most appealing. This can become an expensive fetish, especially if you prefer rubber uniforms and collecting vintage medical equipment. But it doesn't need to be costly, and an improvised gyno chair (bed with lots of pillows stacked up under his/her butt) might be just as effective as that five thousand dollar retro gyno chair you saw on eBay. Be sure that whatever "instruments" you use are sterilized, completely clean, and haven't been used on anyone else, especially if they enter the skin or orifices — you don't want to have a nasty infection (or worse) left behind after your hot fetish encounter. If you're engaging in extreme treatments (see above), learn everything you can about playing safely and seek out supervision for your first few experiments — often you can find an experienced professional dominant that will be happy to safely supervise your play and give you safety pointers (for a fee, of course). Refer to Chapter 10, "Fetish Sex Rules" for basic guidelines and Chapter 11, "Resources," for further reading and websites. Never try something dangerous without professional guidance first. But always use your imagination and have fun!

Medical instruments for your scene might include:
- Neuro wheel, a sharp pointy wheel rolled on the skin used to test nerve response
- Speculum, a duck-billed stretching device used in gynecological examinations
- Stethoscope, used in listening to the heartbeat, lungs, or other body parts
- Tongue depressor, for looking in the mouth
- Latex or nitrile (non-latex) gloves for exams (they feel amazing to wearer and patient alike)

- Enema or douche kits: great for bathroom, humiliation, and age-regression scenes
- Sponges (soft or rough) and towels for bathing
- Bandages, such as Ace or white mummy wrap
- Band-Aids
- Thermometer for oral or rectal temperature-taking; only use rectal thermometers for anal play. You can always substitute fingers, butt toys, or a penis or dildo for a thermometer.
- Adult diapers
- Breast pumps, for milk extraction
- Dental spreaders, basically metal headgear used to hold the mouth open (found at BDSM stores)
- Reflex hammer
- Small flashlight, for examining dark crevasses
- Lubricant
- Forceps, clamps
- Restraints
- Sex toys: penis, clit and nipple pumps, clips and clamps, vibrators, dildos, strap-ons, ball gags
- Medical scissors, for removing clothing and handy for bondage emergencies
- Butcher or medical table paper to spread on your exam table
- A tool tray (can be stainless steel or improvised); a tea tray or nightstand (can be covered with white paper towels and hold your instruments)
- Clipboard, for taking notes (or writing yourself a script to follow if you're nervous)

The World of Adult Baby Play and Diaper Lovers

Age-play fantasies involve one person in the role of regressed age (baby, child, teen) and another person in an adult role, though adult baby fetish, sometimes called infantilism, occupies the baby or infant end of this spectrum. The person playing the younger part is usually the helpless, toddler in age-play fetish, and is often held captive in many ways. Adult baby play (called AB by practitioners and DL for diaper lovers), spans all sexual orientations and genders in its manifestations. In most cases infant play only rarely involves sexual activity. The essence of an adult baby scenario is to create the experience of infancy and usually (though not always) the age period before toilet training. The adult figure can be nurse, mommy, daddy, baby-sitter, teen mother, adoptive parent, other authority figures or relatives or strangers.

AB fetish is one of the most marginalized fetishes in existence, because of the incest overtones, pedophiliac aspects, and distaste that many adults have when considering a masculine man or grown woman becoming aroused by being reduced to a helpless infant, soiling themselves in a diaper. ABs break nearly every taboo in the book simply by what their fetish suggests to outsiders, but in reality AB fetish is a far cry from taboos one might associate with what is in essence intense (and often therapeutic) pampering experiences. People who wish to have sex with children or engage in incest *do*; they do not engage in consensual adult baby play with other adults.

It's common to feel unease upon discovery of your lover's AB fetish. There are a number of things you can do if this is you, or if this brings up bad or difficult feelings about yourself or your relationship. First, read through the first few chapters of this book to understand what a fetish is, how they work, and what they mean—and what to do when you're confused, scared, or unsure about the whole thing. If you're okay with AB play but don't want to "go there" with any incest overtones, you can opt to make your roles unrelated. You can also try being babies together, which might provide insight into what your lover finds so compelling about the fetish. If you totally don't like the idea, try to be accepting of your lover's needs and suggest that an articulate and sympathetic pro domme specializing in AB fetish might be an option, either for sessions or simply for you to talk to and get some questions answered.

But why would someone do this in the first place? Being a baby again is incredibly freeing for the adult tot. They no longer have to think for themselves, which can be a huge relief, even if it's just for an hour. The AB gets the pampering, nurturing, and obsessive love and intimate fussing-over they might need, in a short, concentrated dose. There might be a fetish for a certain feeling that comes with AB play, such as wearing diapers, and anything else only serves to heighten the feeling of comfort or arousal the AB gets from the experience. It's also emotionally intimate and risky; the AB is emotionally exposed and vulnerable. Tension can be resolved by temper tantrums, or just a good hard cry. Here, the AB can do what responsible adults can't, in a very straightforward, honest way: pout, cry, demasculinize (for men), whine, wear frilly things, enjoy passivity and helplessness, and trust someone unconditionally. Being an AB is all feeling and impulse. Maybe being "mommied" just feels good; for many, it's carte blanche permission to just *feel* without being judged, a time to indulge mindlessly without feeling guilty — because if AB is bad, they'll get punished. The scenario of misbehavior, punishment, and forgiveness is often emotionally cathartic and rewarding for both participants. Trust is essential in all AB relationships, but the trust in an AB relationship is deep and absolute.

The online resources for AB play are astounding, and it's overwhelming to see how much detail is put into their resource and shopping websites. In some cases so much detail is put into the terminology and appearance of AB sites, it may take a minute to realize that they're selling adult gear. Often, sissy-boy and -girl play (see my chapter on cross-dressing) overlaps into AB territory and it's typical to see these fetishes in the same forums, and to shop at the same sites for what might be for the fetishist singularly different pursuits.

Things the grownup role can do for the adult baby:
- Dress your adult baby in rubber panties, bib, bonnet, pinafore, and booties
- Feed the AB formula or baby food, or breast-feed
- Diaper the AB: Make a big ritualistic show of "changing" the AB into diapers, complete with baby wipes, powdering, and safety pins
- Keep the AB in diapers the entire time
- Cuddle and pamper the AB; hold and coo, pet and baby-talk, play together with toys
- Play peek-a-boo; put your AB down for a nap; tell nursery rhymes or naptime stories
- Punish the bad baby with a spanking, diapering, or sexual service then offer forgiveness and consolation

- Make the AB soil their diapers; good for ABs that enjoy humiliation, though some will enjoy the sensation for its own sake
- Help or "teach" the AB to masturbate
- Shave the AB; bathe the AB
- Grant the AB permission to have an orgasm
- Administer enemas, temperature-taking, and other minor medical baby maintenance
- Decide if enemas are for health or punishment, and never change your routine
- Toilet-train the AB
- Force them into ruffled panties or other humiliating baby wear — often, forcing the AB into role is an important part of release (always have adult consent first, of course)

Babies Can Play Together

Sometimes you both might want to play as equals, you both might be ABs in a relationship together, you may like to switch roles, or maybe networking has helped you find other ABs to play with. Either way, two or more adult babies can have lots of fun together. You can play with toys together, enjoy messy food (or other substance) play, wrestle, fight, bite, share bottles, and explore each other's bodies and anything else you might enjoy.

AB Gear: Set the Scene

Most items for AB play will be commonly available items at drugstores, supermarkets, and malls, though some items (like adult baby diapers) you'll need to special order from AB websites.

Everyday AB items: baby powder, pacifier, baby lotion, baby toys, rattles, baby safety pins, baby oil.

Special orders, in adult sizes: oversize cribs, high chairs, and playpens; adult-sized diapers (plastic, cotton, or rubber—your AB will have a particular preference); diaper covers; pee pants in plastic or rubber; bib; booties; pajamas with feet; pinafores and petticoats; bonnets; pretty baby dresses or little man outfits; snap-crotch garments such as overalls; bed-wetter pants; bed-wetter sheets

You can use any room in the house for your scene, but if you want to dress it up a little, go for it! Soften any room with a little extra lace or ruffles (pink for girls, blue for boys). Create a nursery by setting up a bed with playful blankets, stuffed animals, and soft lighting. Rattles and nursery rhymes are a nice touch. Don't forget to set out all your AB gear, such as diapers and baby powder, and create a changing station, even if it's just a blanket on the floor.

The adult role—the mommy—may want to set up a punishment area as well, like a stool and wide-paddle hairbrush for spankings. Don't forget to dress the part to emphasize the gap between adult and baby. Think June Cleaver and you're probably on the mark; aprons, girdles, vintage dresses, perfume, makeup, lipstick, long red nails, and even a snap-open nursing bra are all possibilities.

Adult Thumbsucking

A gentle fetish, adult thumbsucking revolves around the reassurance of seeing or experiencing the act of an adult engaging in an often-unconscious childhood comfort ritual. While it may play into sissy or adult baby play, in a large number of adult thumbsucking communities it's not an age-regression fantasy at all, even though the adult thumb-sucker knows that child-related social stigmas come along with the territory. For some it is sexy and highly erotic, for others it's a comforting experience. It's an easy fetish to cater to, though keep in mind that extended years of thumbsucking can cause dental problems and calluses on the thumb or heel of the hand, from teeth.

Everything That Ails You
Thomas Roche

"Poor girl. The doctor won't give you what you need, huh?"

Brenda was tied to the gyno table in the middle of the play floor. Or, more accurately, her lower body was tied to the table. Her upper body, on the contrary, didn't need to be tied to the table—it was bound tightly in a white canvas straitjacket.

She was naked below the waist except for the thick strap of the straitjacket and the secure leather restraints forcing her legs wide open.

Paul, for his part, wore the blue medical scrubs of an intern, an orderly, a male nurse—and the evil expression of an aroused top. The two of them had attracted a small crowd of voyeurs, standing at a respectful distance in a circle around the scene.

"But I know what you need," he growled, his face close to hers. Brenda had been ball-gagged as well as bound, so she couldn't respond verbally; instead, she responded only with the fear in her eyes—and the hot flood between her legs, which she knew Paul would discover momentarily. Because he was unbuckling the crotch strap of the straitjacket.

Brenda tried in vain to close her legs, felt an intense

erotic thrill when she felt the ankle restraints to be secure. In the normal function of the straitjacket, the crotch strap would be an integral part of the restraint—but Brenda was seen to quite securely by the four buckled straps across her back, the tight belt around her waist, the leather straps holding her legs wide open. And the ball gag.

The crotch strap came free, and Brenda moaned behind the gag as Paul's fingers invaded her exposed sex.

"You've been needing it bad," he chuckled, sliding first two and then three fingers into her. She squirmed and struggled as he fingered her in full view of the gathered crowd. "The doctor thinks he can treat you without fucking you, but I know that's the only treatment you need."

Brenda fought violently against her bonds, her arousal mounting as she felt their strength. There was nothing she could do. She could not get away. Her pussy responded with a tightening of the muscles, a raging hunger as she lubricated uncontrollably.

When Paul slid his fingers out of her and reached for the waistband of his scrubs, her pussy went wetter than ever before.

His cock popped out full and hard. He seized a condom from the nearby play bag, tore it with his teeth, and fitted it over his cock with one hand. He positioned himself between her flailing knees and forced them open; the feel of pressure on her legs heightened Brenda's intensifying arousal. When he entered her, all her struggles stopped in an instant, as her back arched with the ecstatic sensations coursing through her.

Paul began to fuck her, his weight pinning her against the table, her struggles beginning anew—harder, now, the pleasure making her surge and buck against him—as his cock plumbed her with long slow thrusts.

"This is what you've been needing," cooed Paul. "This is the treatment that'll cure everything that ails you. Isn't that right?"

Brenda could only respond with a cry from behind the gag, as she reached her climax and her muscles went taut, her struggles stopping in an instant as the pleasure exploded through her. Paul continued fucking her, grunting rhythmically, seeking the particular animalistic sound to his savagery—and finding it just as he reached his own climax, inside her, coming hard as his cock plunged rhythmically into her.

He withdrew with a sigh, looking over his patient, who was now too spent to struggle.

With a smile, he reached over to the play bag. "Of course," he said, snapping on a latex glove and dousing it with lube, "there are *other* treatments that'll help you... "

Brenda began to struggle again, whimpering behind the ball gag as his fingers slid deep inside her again.

Chapter 9
About the Body

The obsessions and fetishes we have for other people's bodies make us understand and recognize the contours of our own bodies in ways we never could before our explorations. Like the Greek god Narcissus, eternally gazing at himself, the wide world of fetish is largely focused inward, on the body — our bodies, others' bodies — and what outrageous and impossible and outlandishly taboo things we can imagine doing with them. Some seem pedestrian, like a fetish for big breasts, but taken to their fetish extremes they become shocking, humorous, arousing, freakish, comforting, and sometimes, confusingly, all of those things at once. Understanding them is only part of the experience; learning to play with them is the fun part.

Breast Fetish

It seems like our entire culture has a breast fetish, but the true breast fetishist sees a pair of boobs—usually a very specific kind, shape, and size—and thinks they are absolutely the most beautiful, sexy, and desirable part of a woman's body. And more than that, they're absolutely required in one way or another for satisfying sexual release. It's a lot more than just liking boobs. It's *needing* them; being obsessed, fascinated, and feeling deeply connected, yet always yearning for them. And wanting to fuck them somehow, of course.

More and more, a significant number of women with naturally overlarge breasts are having them surgically reduced for health and well-being reasons—while simultaneously, a growing number of women around the world—biological females and transgender women—are going the exact opposite direction by having their breasts inflated to comic, vulgar, even physically shocking proportions. As with all fetishes, the outside observer asks why—but not the women getting the enlargements, nor the people (mostly men) who enjoy the augmentation and exaggeration of femininity they represent. Big, huge, overstuffed breasts filled with silicone until they look fit to burst; or gigantic, weighty, physically challenging natural boobs—to a big-tit fetishist, this is heaven.

But not all big tit fetishists like fake breasts, as many a fetishist has exacting preferences on just what it is they like—and what they like to do—with big boobs. Fake or real, big nipples or small, hard or soft, torpedoes or funbags...they're the highlight of any sexual encounter, and are often an absolute requirement on any sex partner for the big-boob fetishist.

Tit-fucking and smothering are the two most popular

ways for the big-boob sexual encounter to be enjoyed. Tits can be squeezed together to create a soft chasm for a penis, providing tits to squeeze and a terrific view of the owner's boobs and facial expression for the person doing the fucking. Smothering can happen in a variety of positions. Facedown, he can press his face into a world of boob. From below he can surrender to breathlessness and helplessness. If he kneels and she sits, he can lean face-forward into happiness while he masturbates.

Not Naturally Endowed?

Surgery isn't your only option. A trip to Victoria's Secret might surprise you—new bra technology can create some startling real-life morphs on your very own chest, making a B-cup look like a D, or more. Also, don't be afraid to check out the trans resources in the back of this book for breast-enhancement tricks; sometimes a huge, real-feeling (but carefully constructed) rack inside a tight sweater might be just what the doctor ordered.

Big boobs can also be used to taunt and tease him. Give him a taste; rub them all over his body; use his hands as you would your own and squeeze and rub until he can't take it anymore—of course, all while dressed in something appropriately tight, revealing, and with a nice scented or flavored lotion in your ample cleavage. Tight white cotton tops, tube tops, it's all good, and in fact a huge bra or any other breast-specific garment might be an excellent sex toy all on its own. Big boobs can be licked, sucked, set on faces, heads, penises, feet, even ordinary household objects, or used as pillows for the boob owner or fetishist. They can be decorated; clipped; clamped; festooned with rope, ribbons and bows; nursed; and suspended with chains or anything else you can imagine to wrap around or hang off them. Big nipples can be pumped even bigger with suction cups, breast pumps, and sex toys, and can be wrapped or even used to hang pretty ornaments.

Not on the Itty Bitty Titty Committee?

No big deal—a trip to a decent lingerie store will help you find bras one or several sizes smaller than your natural size. Strap 'em down, flatten them out with sports bras, or even wrap them with an Ace bandage under your clothes to give the illusion of flatness. And after you have your fun, remove the wrap and—boing! Back to bouncy bliss.

Some tit fetishists wouldn't go near a fake breast if it were the last one on Earth (okay, maybe if it were the *last* one). But there are purists in every fetish genre, and some despise the artificial, just as a significant number of breast fetishists prefer the small end of the spectrum. Teacup titties, tiny boobies, small breasts, flat-chested women—they're no less rare than the huge-boobed babes, but still just as lust inducing for the small-tit lover. Most of what the big-tit fetishist likes can be adapted to suit the tastes of a flat-chest fetishist; tit-fucking a flat chest feels incredible, especially if aided by lubricant and hands, and rubbing tiny tits—smothering his face from above, below, or seated—might produce surprising results. Small breasts and tiny nipples can be decorated, and put through various types of bondage and torture as well. Nipples can be enlarged with pumps to hold clamps and clips, twine and even rope, or can be decorated with a rope harness.

Butt Fetish

I know you're thinking "Bootylicious" and you're right; big asses sit in the royal throne of this fetish. Think of the cartoon artist Robert Crumb and his obsession with gigantic bubble butts and you're on the right track—watching them walk, move, sit on things, sit on his face, crush him, smother him, and even used as a seat for riding around on his Amazonian creations. While some fantasies the big-butt fetishist may have might not be actually physically possible, it's fun to play around with the butt fetishist, and if you're naturally endowed you have a terrific sex toy right in your back pocket(s). Butt and leg fetishes often go "hand in hand," and a nice trick is to put your lover in charge of rubbing lotion into your legs and ass as regular maintenance. Similarly, panty fetish and ass fetish are often combined. And yes, anal sex and butt play are likely high on the to-do list for fun and games with your butt-lover (see Chapter 10, "Fetish Sex Rules," for anal-play tips and safety hints).

Don't Have a J-Lo?

You don't need to get butt implants (though some people do). Check the resources chapter for trans solutions for flat butts and don't be embarrassed—just give yourself a bubble butt and don't go bare-assed! There are oodles of panties, shorts and girdles made for women and men alike to give the illusion of bootie; use this ass technology to your advantage and give your ass fetishist something to drool over.

Foot and Leg Fetish

Toe, heel, arch, socks, shoes, and toenails are all elements for foot fetish fun, but they have to be pretty, look a certain way, or be of a particular size (small, large) or proportion. Often, for a foot fetishist it might be the one thing that makes or breaks what makes someone (usually female) attractive. Many foot fetishists enjoyed the Paris Hilton porn video *1 Night in Paris* until the moment they saw her feet—her long, bony feet and articulated toes were a huge turn-off to this fetish contingent. But it's not just looking at—or having —nice feet that gets the foot fetishist off; it's also what can be done with feet that can be a huge turn-on. Pedicures, foot-fucking, toe-sucking, foot massage, crotch-rubbing, and even performing acts with the feet and toes (like smoking or masturbating) are all possibilities with a foot lover. Shoes, socks and nylons, stockings or pantyhose may also be an essential component—dressing them up properly is always important. It's quite common for foot and leg fetishes to be combined.

If you find yourself with a foot fetishist, the first thing you should do is get a professional pedicure, stat! A pro will condition, massage, clean, soften, and primp your feet so they look their beautiful best, and you'll feel confident when your lover handles them, knowing that your feet are perfect in appearance, feel, and scent. Maintain your pretty feet and make foot care part of your daily regimen with lotions, scrubs, and regular maintenance—better yet, assign this maintenance to your lover. Some may like it if you erotically command or force them to take care of your feet.

Seduce, tease, and fuck your lover with your feet at every opportunity. When they're watching, slip a foot out of your shoe, even in public, just to give them a look to savor for later. Rub your foot on their foot, their leg, or even their crotch through their clothing for a desired effect. Make them suck or lick your toes, while they touch themselves or you masturbate them. When it comes time for foot-fucking, press your foot on their crotch; drizzle lube or oil over your feet or their genitals and rub it in with your feet. If your lover is male, make a hollow with your arches to create a space for him to fuck, and hold your feet together with your hands to keep it tight (or let him control your feet). Make him come on your feet; make him lick it off.

Ear Fetish

Yes, there is a fetish for every body part. But don't think that ear fetish is just another parts obsession—no, ear fetish, though more popular in Japan than anywhere else upon this writing, is about particular shapes of ears and watching things happen to the ears. Usually, the things ear fetishists like to see are cleaning, the insertion and removal of ear plugs, ear piercing, and of course pictures of very nice ears. Some may like to smell, lick, or rub the ears (usually of pretty girls). Sites devoted to ear fetish typically have galleries of ears, with no other body parts or pornographic content.

Nose Fetish, or Pinocchia

Big noses, natural or computer morphed, are the hallmark of the Pinocchia fetish, named for the fondness of making the noses of pretty women grow, like in the classic tale "Pinocchio," Unlike ear fetish, Pinocchia is typically a fairly sexually explicit fetish, and it's common to see porn photos used in the morphs—though not always. Celebrities are popular candidates for nose morph, and the morphs are not always about lengthening of the nose; just a larger than normal nose might be enough for the

Violet Blue

fetishist to get a twinge of arousal, and someone who
morphs a picture might just make a tiny nose into a bul-
bous honker—because they think it looks hot. This is a
bonus if you have a big nose, though because this fetish is
typically an image-centered fixation it's no big deal if your
nose is smaller than ones your lover likes. Just help them
find more pictures! Nose bondage, where the nose is
pulled with rope, pressed with leather straps, or creative-
ly bound and pulled with nose hooks, is another Japanese
import that has been recently getting more attention in the
United States. Consult bondage books for clever nose
bondage ideas if this is your cup of tea, and never play
with nose bondage in any way that might restrict oral
breathing, especially if the submissive has allergies or a
stuffy nose.

Hair (Trichophilia)

Extremely long hair, head shaving, hirsuteness (body
hair), and unshaven women populate the most trafficked
highways of hair fetish. Hair fetish manifests in many
ways—from a sexual preference for European (unshaven)
women, all the way to ultra-hairy porn, or instant arousal
at the thought of watching a woman get her head shaved.

Body hair lovers typically fall into two camps: the
Hair to Stay crowd and bear-lust. *Hair to Stay* is a magazine and Website devoted to "lovers of naturally hairy
women" and features erotic and explicit photos of very
hairy women showing off armpit, genital and leg hair,
and hair growing everywhere. A "bear" is typically a
heavy gay male with full facial hair and copious body
hair, with a subculture and terminology too enormous to
cover here—though for our purposes we can refer to bear-

lovers as someone of any gender who loves and fetishizes hairy men.

Bald fetish is a fairly (though not always) straight-male fetish, in which a man enjoys seeing long or copious hair shaved completely off — though some may simply get hot at the sight, feel, or picture of a sexy bald woman. The act of shaving a woman's head is possibly the pinnacle of an erotic encounter for a few bald fetishists, and because you can only shave long hair once every few months (or more) it might be a "once in a while" fetish. If you have no intention of shaving your head but you know your lover is into shaving, let them shave the underside of your hair so it's not obvious or entrust them in shaving other parts of your body (see the shaving section in Chapter 7, "Cross-Dressing and Sissies," for tips). But it might just be the shaved head that does it for them, though don't despair; let them indulge in their fantasies by CGI morphs, Photoshop, or the several bald fetish communities online.

Long hair lovers enjoy the sight, smell, and feel of extremely long hair, and may like to masturbate with, brush, comb, or wash the hair. It's not uncommon for the long-hair fetishist to steal clandestine touches of long hair in public places, though they should be reminded that this is nonconsensual — especially if the fetishist considers it a sexual act. Long-hair fetish groups are a great resource.

Fingernails

Short fingernails and the way they feel, sure — but the heavyweights in nail fetish are those who love extremely long fingernails. Shockingly long, and typically female and painted. For these fetishists, the fingernails are the ultimate representation of strength and femininity, even if to the casual onlooker it seems that the owners of these talons might not be able to perform many everyday functions. Long red fingernails are the queen of this fetish and just the sight—or threat—that red nails pose or represent can get nail fetishist' worked into an erotic frenzy. In some scenarios the nails play an important visual part of the sexual encounter; in other cases it's typical to see fetish galleries devoted to images only of the models' hands—seldom their faces or any pornographic content. Fingernail fetish stories include being pinched and scratched by specific types of fingernails.

Inflation

Body inflation specifically relates to seeing, experiencing, or morphing images of body parts (usually genitals, lips, or breasts) inflated by external pumping or saline injections. Penis, nipple, and clit pumps create a vacuum of air around the area of desired increase, and removal of air through pumping causes blood to rush into the sealed-off area and grows the part within the cylinder or seal. This should always be done slowly, as the effect can be similar to that of a hickey—where capillaries break and leave bruising—and can pave the way to serious nerve damage. Because of this, you should never pump anything for longer than 10 minutes without a rest, and you should always go slowly. The inflation from pumping is temporary, despite the claims of penis-enlargement companies, whose techniques can lead to permanent nerve damage and ED. The pumped organ is bigger and highly responsive to erotic stimulation (it feels great), though especially with the penis you'll find that it's certainly bigger but no harder—you'll have a big, soft-ish dick that's fun to play with.

Saline injection of body parts can increase their size to comic (or frightening) proportions, and the effect is temporary, until the saline absorbs into the body. Just as with pumping, go slow and don't overdo so as to avoid nerve damage, and never try it on your own or without supervision from an expert (usually a pro domme)—at least until you're totally capable of safely playing with saline and needles. An accidental injection of air into your bloodstream can kill you.

Rubber inflation fetish (inflatophilia) is where the person is inside something that's inflated around them or has inflation tubes put pressure against (or inside) them. Inflation might require the complete sensory deprivation of the participant and even immersion into water before their "suit" is inflated; or, they might want to be sealed in a vacuum bag (with air tubes, of course). The resulting feeling varies in description from person to person, in some cases creating a deliriously womb-like and comfortable space, a terrifying asphyxiation fantasy, and erotic helplessness. Pressure outfits and garments are inflated with squeeze-balls to put pressure (usually erotic) on various body parts, though the inflated garment might be part of a full suit or transformation persona complete with mask (as part of a gender-transformation outfit). Sometimes items are placed in the mouth, anus, or vagina and inflated for feelings of fullness, stretching, submission, and obvious erotic stimulation.

Scars

Scar-tissue fetishes range from the accidental to the self-inflicted, and have different meanings for each individual.

The places where the scars melt into the skin may hold special appeal, or it may be the acts of violence upon the skin and their evidence that create an erotic spark for the fetishist. Body modification that includes scarification crosses into this realm, whereas some people who get decorative (or "tribal") scarring for aesthetic purposes may or may not get an erotic charge out of the process or results. Of all the morphing fetishes, this one is easiest to re-create in real life harmlessly. Visit a costume store or online Halloween shop to find a variety of fake scars you can use to surprise and treat your scar fetishist with.

Pregnancy (Maiesiophilia) and Lactation (Galactophilia)

A fetish with such a significant population that it occupies its own porn genre, pregnancy and lactation fetish, like big-boob fetish, is so mainstreamed in many ways that it's even been acted out in popular media. The episode of the TV show *Angel* in which one character becomes pregnant and comes to full term has been hotly debated on pregnancy/lactation websites as to whether the storyline was penned by a fellow fetishist. Same with the episode of *Malcolm in the Middle* in which the husband attempts to fatten up his pregnant wife because he finds it irresistibly arousing—another common fantasy among pregnancy fetishists.

These are playful and insightful ways into looking at a fetish that is often confused by outsiders as having to do with malice toward women or interest in pedophilia, which is far from the reality of pregnancy fetish. This is also very different than fat fetish (see next entry). People into this fetish (and there's a significant gender equality here) don't want babies or birth; they love the sight of giant bellies and breasts swollen with milk, and there are a number of specifics tailor-made for each fetishist's fixation. First, she can't be "too big" (though a few people get off on the out-of-control swelling concept) or not pregnant enough. There's a slight resemblance to inflation (see above), but what typifies the fetish tends to be the sheer impossibility of many common scenarios. Being several months overdue, carrying around practically a litter, forever pregnant, pregnancy so rapid it can be watched, and lactation: leaky breasts, squirting breast milk, the woman drinking her own milk out of giant breasts, and nursing adult men (not adult babies, though there is crossover with this fetish as well—see Chapter 8, "Medical Play and Adult Babies").

Fat Fetish

If you just read this and thought, "Oh, I'm kinda fat. This could be fun!" chances are good you're wrong—most people reading this, even if overweight, don't qualify as "babe" status for the fat fetishist. The fat fetishist is a bit more than a "chubby chaser" (though this term is affectionately used in fat fetish communities); rather, the fat fetishist prefers the seriously obese lover—typically fat women in the 300–400-pound range, though there's equal play in all genders and orientations. *Real fat*, as in people gawk and stare when the fat person walks by, and that too turns on the fat fetishist. Unlike many fetishes that primarily focus on images and computer-generated alterations, fat fetish gets a lot of real-life action as this is a fairly well-populated country with lots of enthusiasts with a variety of angles on just what turns them on about fat girls.

"FAs," or fat admirers, comprise a huge subculture, and much celebratory sex and many rewarding relationships are found between FAs and people in the fat acceptance movement (such as NAAFA and excellent books such as *Fat! So?* by Marilyn Wann).

This is a huge (no pun) subculture, with plenty of porn available, a wide lexicon of terms and oodles of communities, books, magazines, websites, and more. There's quite a bit of fantasy here for sure, and you'll find celebrity fat morph sites, but many fat fetishists prefer to rollick and play in the flesh—literally—of their lovers. They find the limited mobility of their lovers attractive, and sex for the fat fetishist is an adventure of insertion into as many billowing, lubricated folds as possible. They enjoy the clothes worn by their huge paramours, and some fantasize about their lovers growing larger and larger—prompting many support groups for women who have ended their relationships with "feeders" due to health and emotional reasons. Feeders are just that: They fixate on increasing the size of their fat lovers through feeding. There are outspoken feedees who derive sexual pleasure from being fed for the purposes of fattening up, and this is by no means an exclusively fat-submissive fetish; many fat female dominants consider themselves powerful giantesses, looking for skinny little sex partners to dominate and crush—and to feed them.

It's healthy to love fat people, and fat fetish is satisfying for many people—but fattening someone up has negative health consequences, and being "morbidly obese" (while hot for some) can be a life-threatening health condition and can shorten the lifespan of your fat lover. There's no harm in gaining a few pounds for your sweetie and they're easily shed if you decide you don't like it.

Conversely, you can always play around with fat suits (available at costume stores) if you want to entertain fantasy fat-fetish scenarios.

Chastity, Virginity, and Sexual-Initiation Scenarios

Having your sexuality — specifically your genitals — under the complete control of another person is a very common fantasy, but when fantasy becomes fetish and more fantasies evolve from the fetish...well, you have fetishes that revolve around chastity and virginity and what happens when another person lays claim to your parts.

Chastity play — in which male or female genitals are put literally under lock and key by a dominant partner — is a staple in BDSM play. But chastity fetish is when the scene revolves around the chastity device and sexual servitude related specifically to the device. Chastity devotees can purchase a number of toys on BDSM websites (such as JT's Stockroom — see Chapter 11, "Resources"), but many prefer to make, create, and invent their own devices that maintain the sexual unavailability of the wearer. Many devices are created to punish the wearer upon arousal, specifically male wearers, and to make wearers sexually available to whoever might want to satisfy their whims. Some have cock cages, some anal-insertive devices; others completely restrict access to genitalia and require humiliating predicaments during which the wearer must relieve themselves. Chastity belts and cages might be pretty or simply functional in appearance; or the more medieval the better, metal and leather being commonly used construction materials.

Chastity belts were traditionally used to maintain the fidelity and/or virginity of the wearer, and to restrict masturbation. But restriction leads to release, and here's where we cross over into virginity and sexual-initiation fetishes. These aren't underage fantasies, though reliving our own first fumbling experiences can sometimes be hot, healing, and playful. Rather, it's the desire to be the "first," to deflower, to sexually teach—or to be the one who "learns" how to masturbate from a more experienced friend, or has their "cherry popped." Sure there's a "cult of youth" aspect to this fetish, but one could argue that as politically incorrect as it may seem (or as hot as the fantasy is for many people), a good many religions have what many might deem a fairly unhealthy virginity fetish themselves. Think about it.

Wet and Messy Play

WAM, or wet and messy fetish, is one of the most carefree and playful fetishes around—though for the person who gets instantly hard or wet seeing sexy people slather themselves with wet and gooey substances, or sit in pastries or cheesecake, it's a serious...pleasure. Sploshing (as it's called by many participants) is the smearing, pouring, sitting in, and accidental spilling of food, liquids, or other messy substances, ranging from whipped cream to mud and everything in between. If you think this is weird, I highly recommend you try it, at least once. There's something so hilariously playful about pouring chocolate syrup over one's head, and so undeniably sexy about a pair of breasts smeared with sticky sweet substances, begging for a rub, a lick, or cleanup. And wet and messy clothing tends to get pretty revealing.

Messy-play fans, like their many fetish counterparts, have pretty specific tastes when it comes to what they like in a messy scene. Dirt and/or salty items might be a disgusting no-no; for these aficionados only sweet syrups might suffice. Or, chocolate might look too much like feces to be a turn-on, whereas an adult schoolgirl sitting on cupcakes (or squishing them between her feet) might bring him close to spontaneous ejaculation. Books, websites, pay porn sites, magazine,s and online communities contribute to make this a huge fetish, with lots of happy participants—with likely sizeable laundry and plumbing bills.

Smoking (Capnolagnia)

One of the fetishes that—when done right—is one of the sexiest things to watch, smoking is typically the most underserved and poorly executed fetishes around. Smoking fetish is just that: watching someone (usually a pretty girl with perfect lipstick) smoke. The smoker might smoke during sexual situations, while the fetishist masturbates, or may demonstrate a variety of smoking techniques and means of sexily blowing the smoke—into another person's mouth, onto body parts, or with an air of disinterest, off into nowhere. Many porn companies and websites have tried to produce smoking porn, but as with most fetishes, their lack of understanding about what makes smoking sexy for the viewer results in poor and uninteresting smoking videos. The best erotic smoking videos are made by porn director Andrew Blake, and they feature mostly girl-girl scenarios. If your lover gets hot watching someone smoke, there's no need to pick up a deadly habit (or make your bedroom smell) just to satisfy his or her needs. Buy a pack of organic or imported ultra-light cigarettes, a nice lighter, and maybe a cigarette holder (or several), and fake-smoke your way through your encounter. Take a puff, hold it in your mouth (don't inhale), and slowly expel it with a puff of air from your lungs. Experiment and take your time with your smoking ritual; often it's all the ritual, preparation and time taken during the smoking that allows the fetishist to fully enjoy their experience.

Amputees (Apotemnophilia) and Devotees (Acrotomophilia)

Amputee fetish is one of the more trafficked fetishes when anyone brings up a fetish for shock value (along with human ponies, wet and messy play and fat fetish), and it has its own communities, porn sites, terminology and hard-to-find magazines. While certainly a taboo fetish, much of amputee fetish lives in the form of computer-morphed imagery, called ES or electronic surgery pics. These include anything from fantasy scenarios to found pictures of ordinary women passed off as the "real" thing, and celebrity-amputee-fantasy CGI morphs. In amputee fetish, there are generally the amputees themselves (or wannabes, who may act out their desires by binding to appear publicly as an amputee) and devotees, those who are fans of finger, body-part, and limb amputation.

Much of what comprises amputee fetish fantasies is simply seeing the amputation site, but also what would happen sexually with the amputee in the absence of whatever part is missing. Some are not excited as much by the loss of the limbs or surgery, but rather the way the amputee moves without their lower legs (also called 2AK, or "double above the knee"). The limblessness may not need to be caused by accident or surgery and may have begun at birth. Participants claim erotic surprise and excitement at the powerful "wholeness" of the person who is definitely human but also somehow supernatural in their abilities.

Conversely, some amputee devotees have elaborate caretaking fantasies about their lovers; there are also erotic interests to be found here in the associated equipment, like prosthesis and creating fantasy prosthesis. There are a significant number of amputees who are very excited to find a subculture of sexual interest, as they no doubt do not stop becoming sexual people after having limbs removed for whatever reasons. Of course, a number of amputees find eroticization of their stumps offensive, to say the least. And while there is a cultural fascination with obsessive amputee-devotee relationships where parts are removed in a sinister fashion, this type of relationship is impossible to find documentation of outside of Internet claims.

Bodily Fluids: Blood (Hematolagnia), Defecation (Coprophilia), Spitting, Urination (Urolagnia), Vomit (Ephebophilia), and Expectoration

Erotic expectoration fetish includes sneezing, coughing, nose-blowing, and spitting. In general, the most erotic part of these oft-involuntary fluid expulsions is the facial expressions or sounds associated with the acts. Many sneeze and cough fetishists like the orgasmic look of helplessness or surprise that precedes and follows a sneeze or cough. Some fetishists, though not all, enjoy fantasizing about what might have caused the cough, such as smoking, a cold, emphysema, or choking. Erotic outlets for cough fetishists are smoking forums, because they can find people describing their smoking coughs at delicious length.

Scat fans enjoy watching sexy people relieve themselves — they're into pooping, and this fetish is another all-gender, all-orientation equal-opportunity obsession, despite popular conceptions about it occurring between men and girls. It's often a voyeur's fetish, though there are plenty of people who enjoy not just the sight (and what they associate with it: intimacy, taboo, revulsion, humiliation) but also the sound, the smell, the feel and yes, the taste of feces. Possible elements may include toilets and bathrooms, "accidents" and soiled underwear, purposeful or forced oral ingestion, and unwashed anuses. The most important thing to understand when it comes to scat play are the practicalities, namely that ingestion of feces in many instances can give the consumer Hepatitis A — by all means, if you prefer to play this way, do get your Hepatitis shots and follow up on them; you're also at risk for a number of bacterial diseases and any parasites that your pooping friend may be carrying. And follow safer sex precautions by never engaging in coprophagy if you have any cuts or sores in your mouth or before or after brushing your teeth (which opens up tiny cuts in your gums), or you will be susceptible to viruses as well.

Pee play and pissing fetish has become quite mainstream in porn, and while you should follow the same safer-sex guidelines as stated above, urine is sterile when it leaves the body and thus safer to play with and swallow. Pissing fetish involves watching, listening, being a human toilet or target, being peed on for pleasure and/or ownership, taboo or humiliation, watching pretty girls (and boys) have "accidents," urination during sex (not to be confused with female ejaculation), seeing sexy people get peed on, and surprise encounters.

Human Furniture (Forniphilia)

Put simply, forniphilia is the art of using bondage to turn humans into furniture—functional furniture. Of course, this furniture is more than a human table on which to set your drink; you can also fuck the table whenever you feel like it, as forniphilia is steeped in BDSM, sexual ownership, and the rites and rituals of bondage. People— usually women—are made into chairs, lamps, tables, set into dinner tables, and in the more elaborate configurations found at the celebrated forniphilia site House of Gord (houseofgord.com), working sprinkler systems, car bumpers, utility items and every imaginable household, human-size inanimate object. The keys here are bondage, aesthetics, and sexual availability of the subject. Before jumping into the complex world of forniphilia, experiment first *without* bondage, observe and study House of Gord, and familiarize yourself with safety in bondage techniques; this isn't bondage for beginners.

Giantesses (Macrophilia), Trampling, and Being Crushed

The macrophile is into a bit more than big women; think more like fantasies about women the size of the Statue of Liberty and you'll get the idea. Purely a fantasy fetish seen mostly in CGI and morph artwork (often featuring celebrities), giantess fetish is the intense desire to see perfectly proportioned women who can lounge against skyscrapers like they were easy chairs—though in this fetish the women are often sexually predatory, have animalistic urges, anger easily, and are readily able to swallow, vaginally, or anally insert the viewer or crush him with finger, ass, or high heel. Most of the giantesses in this fetish realm are digitally manipulated to look super-tall, while the males in these fantasies are equally made to shrink to the size of a peanut; foot fetish gets a nice representation here as well, as many of the small men wind up being smooshed under big, beautiful feet. With a giantess lover, it's easy to role-play the part of a giantess (see Chapter 4, "The Heart of Fetish: Role-Play") and create custom giantess, sexual crushing, and smothering scenarios.

Trampling is similar to the giantess fetish in that the observer likes to see women—usually in high heels—trampling or walking on small men, though sometimes this crosses over into pretty discomforting territory and the viewer enjoys real-life bug-crushing. People into trampling (and by extension, crushing) might like to watch, or pretend to be the hapless creature being crushed. Because of a case involving a man who created and sold videos depicting small animals being crushed—he was arrested on animal cruelty charges—in 1998 the U.S. Congress banned interstate trafficking of crush videos. In 2002, Britain followed suit, sending four crush video makers (one male, three females) to prison.

Balloons and Looners

"Looners" have a number of ways they like to get off. They might like pictures of clothed women popping balloons, to hump large balloons until they pop, to watch sexy people blow up balloons, or desire to be encased in a balloon. Often, as with coughing and sneezing, the look on a woman's face when a balloon pops might be the one thing that gets them off the most. Fortunately this is one of the easier fetishes to play with; a trip to the party store yields a whole evening's fun— surprise your looner with a balloon-popping striptease! A nice gallery can be found at loonerz.com.

Human Mannequins, Statues (Agalmatophilia), and Robots

This is for people who become aroused by machinery, machines that are sex toys, or people who are secretly machines. They may become a machine, or get aroused when you are revealed to be a machine (humanized machines may fall under the "human doll" category). This is an imagery-driven fetish, but sex machines that vibrate and penetrate (such as the expensive Sybian) can be purchased online. See fuckingmachines.com and sybian.com. In human machine fetish, the role of inanimate humanoid can be played by you or your lover. Mannequins and human dolls can be dressed and undressed, positioned, admired, and used sexually without protest.

Midgets

Midgets, dwarves, and smaller-than-average people are all principle parts of this fetish. This may include watching midgets engaged in sexual situations such as in porn, looking at images, role-playing midget sex, or having different types of sexual encounters with midgets.

Tickling

Some might like to be tickled, have particular parts of their bodies (like feet) tickled, enjoy tickling a sexy person, like to watch sexy people tickle each other, or like tickling pushed to the limits with tears and involuntary urination. Many who like to be tickled become very aroused and will want to masturbate, and you can restrain them and give them a hand job while you tickle or any other sexually devious scenario you think they might like—just tickle them while you do it. When they just like to watch, you can watch tickling videos, talk dirty, and have role-play tickling scenes, or momentarily tickle a friend while your lover watches. For a fun and sexy video featuring naughty adult schoolgirls tickling each other to tears, see Maria Beatty's *Converted to Tickling*.

Sleeping

Simply put, a dormant body is quite enticing. A sleep fetish is when the fetishist gets turned on by being sexually used while they're asleep; someone who gets aroused watching others sleep (clothed or not), or have fantasies about having sex with someone who is asleep. Sleep porn typically involves a sleep catalyst and setup for a believable sleep sex situation, such as the pretty girl who hits her head, or the baby-sitter who gets slipped a sleeping drug; yes, this is a nonconsensual fantasy, pure and simple, and requires the "sleeper" to playact and feign unconsciousness. This is an easy and fun one to play with—good luck trying to stay "asleep" when you're turned on.

Carrying or "Lift and Carry"

Images of sexually attractive people being carried, as in across a threshold or in states of injury, duress or sleep, are at the center of this fetish. Sex may not even be a significant part of the fetish; the act of carrying is generally the most important and poignant element of the scenario. It's sometimes an essential part of sleep fetish, though images of girls lifting and carrying each other, women carrying men and vice-versa are also a huge turn-on for LC fetishists.

Necrophilia

I've heard two very different lectures on necrophilia for human sexuality students through the course of my tenure lecturing to students about fetishes.. In one, it was clear that the woman giving the lecture clearly believed that necrophilia fetish was an urban legend and offered no information about what to say when faced with actual questions about it. The other, given by a good friend and sex-education colleague, was so packed with practical factual information that I wondered (and still do) just how interested he really is in necrophilia. Needless to say, it was an excellent lecture.

So while there are two camps about necrophilia as a fetish—whether real or not, or the fetishist wants to imagine their fantasy made reality—it's essential to take a look at what the core elements of the sexual experience are for the fetishist, so they can be adeptly used as a sex toy for fun and games. Because what I realized after putting the two lectures together in my head was that taking some fetishes too seriously is a discredit to the human sexual imagination, and that yes, there is a sense of humor underlying every sexual fetish that may appear as morbid or "wrong" to the outsider. And the fetishist knows that. But what they want is more information to make their fantasy as real as possible.

Necrophilia fetish is very similar to sleep fetish: The sexualized person is immobile, helpless, unable to see, hear, feel, or most importantly, judge the person having their way with them. Playing with necro scenes can involve vampire undertones. The scene can be decorated and costumed in Victorian or goth detail, might take place at accident sites (e.g., natural or overdose deaths at home), or might have the added medical fetish of taking place in a morgue or hospital (improvised at home, of course). Body coolness can be increased with a cool shower or bath before play, and makeup can add the sexy pallor of the undead your lover yearns for. Actual sex with a corpse isn't recommended for the obvious reasons of legality, nonconsensuality, and violation, but also because embalming fluid is highly carcinogenic and will burn your skin severely should you come into contact with skin or orifices soaked in it—which most corpses surely are. And one burned penis is enough to kill any fantasy vs. reality argument, once and for all.

Chapter 10
Fetish Sex Rules

Fetish Sex Rule #1: Get Clear Consent From Anyone Involved

Friends and acquaintances might seem like appealing fantasy fetish-sex partners, and in many cases, the fetish revolves around a total stranger and this is what holds the appeal. But if you don't have clear permission to engage in your fetish with someone—anyone—then what you are doing is nonconsensual, and depending on what, who, where, and how you're enjoying your fetish, it's probably illegal. Plus, involving someone in your sexual fetish without permission just isn't cool.

But what if you know the person? There's a lot to consider before you approach someone you know. The risks are obvious—rejection, loss of friendship, sometimes more if the person is someone you work with or see on a regular basis. Consider absolutely off limits people whose workplaces you frequent, like coffee shops, unless you absolutely know you already have an amorous outside-work relationship blooming and everyone is clear about boundaries. If you're unsure for any reason, don't proceed. As with any sexual relationship, you stand to lose someone as a friend if the relationship, or the suggestion of one, isn't well received.

With someone you know, look for clues that indicate their interest in your fetish. But even if you know they're into you, it may still be beyond their friendship boundaries to change their friendship with you. Find out. Tell him or her what you are interested in and see how they react. Directness is scary at first, but it's your most helpful tool. Being honest about fantasies, expectations, concerns and boundaries is your insurance against miscommunication, mishaps, trust issues, and can keep you from getting involved with someone incompatible. Consent is a necessary tool when playing with strangers or someone new. With *anyone*. If someone or something cannot look you in the eye and expressly, specifically say "I want to" then do not proceed, even if it's something as seemingly innocent as a clandestine stroke of his or her hair.

Negotiating your desires can be a matter of quick conversation over drinks, or can take days or weeks of getting to know each other. There might be a lot to discuss, such as fantasy details, rules and limits, safe words, what type of sex is okay, safer sex (who's got condoms, etc.), spending the night (or hour, or weekend) together, who pays for the rubber panties or hotel room, and more. You'll talk about this stuff as the event progresses as well, and everyone has the option of changing their minds as things unfold. Don't ever make a move until the other person clearly states that they're okay with exactly what you want to do, and don't be afraid to make them restate your desires clearly.

Just as you should never touch anyone without asking permission first, don't ever make any assumptions about the person (or people) you've invited into your sex lives. He or she not only needs equal affection, communication and consideration (and orgasms!), but they also might be experiencing a range of feelings. Don't let them feel left out, but while you're thinking about their needs, conversely be aware of what they want from you. If they're cold toward you, don't go any further, and if you sense indifference or ambivalence about your fetish, boundaries or feelings, don't play with them.

Illegal Fetishes

A number of fetishes are illegal for varying reasons in different countries, states, jurisdictions and counties. Consult your local laws. Never engage in illegal activities. These fetishes are known to be illegal (if practiced), everywhere:

- Necrophilia: sexual attraction to corpses. In this book, necrophilia is considered a fantasy sex act
- Necrozoophilia: sexual attraction to the corpses or killings of animals (also known as necrobestiality)
- Frotteurism: sexual arousal through rubbing one's body against a nonconsenting stranger in public
- Telephone scatologia: being sexually aroused by making obscene telephone calls
- Zoophilia: sexual acts with animals, or bestiality

Fetish Sex Rule #2: Know and Practice Safer Sex

Know how to avoid catching and unwittingly spread disease and infections, to protect yourself and those you care about. Don't enact any self-destructive tendencies on innocent strangers by being ignorant about STDs. I'm using the term "safer" instead of "safe" to indicate the practice of using barriers and proper lubrication to prevent injury and the spread of disease. That's because barriers (such as condoms) are not one hundred percent foolproof in protecting each participant from contracting an STD or virus from sexual contact. There are many factors involved in every sexual encounter, and each party takes and assesses risks in each situation—risks including making judgment calls in the heat of the moment. This is especially true when you're in a couple trying out a threesome, sex parties, swinging, or having sex with strangers in any context. So "safer" indicates that safe-sex knowledge and accessories like condoms are safer than nothing.

Always use plenty of water-based lubricant, even if you don't think you need it. Sex feels incredible on slicked-up parts, and latex absorbs moisture, making condoms more susceptible to breakage. Remember, rubber fetishists, what breaks a condom will damage your favorite rubber gimp hood. For condoms, a drop of lube in the tip gives more pleasure and sensation to both the wearer and the recipient of penetration—once you try it, you'll never go back. Water-based lubes are friendly on the vaginal ecosystem, won't break latex (any tiny bit of oil will destroy latex almost instantly), and come in hypo-allergenic formulas. Avoid lubes with the detergent Nonoxynol-9, which causes abrasions on mucous membranes (ouch), and sensitive women should avoid lubes with glycerin, a sugar that contributes to yeast infections.

Condoms

A condom is a snug sheath that unrolls onto a penis or sex toy. Available in latex and polyurethane, in dozens of sizes, colors and flavors. Animal-skin condoms do not prevent the spread of some viruses. Use condoms for fellatio, vaginal and anal sex, and for covering sex toys that are made of porous materials, or when you want to share a sex toy. Change condoms for different sex partners, different sex toys, and different orifices — something used anally should be covered with a condom before being inserted orally or vaginally. Do not use anything containing oils of any kind where latex condoms may come in contact; however, polyurethane condoms may be used with oils.

Dental Dams

Thin squares of latex or polyurethane used as a barrier for cunnilingus and rimming. Lubricate the genitals, place the dam on top, keep a good hold on the dam, and lick to your heart's content. They're available in a few flavors and colors, and in a jam you can use plastic wrap or a condom cut open and laid flat.

Gloves

Use latex or non-latex gloves for touching anyone's genitals. They protect against germs from your hands going onto genitals, can protect your hands from picking up viruses or germs, and make hands a smooth surface free of jagged nails or scratchy calluses.

Fingercots

Tiny condoms made of latex that unroll over a finger to create a sterile surface. Great for on-the-go escapades.

Safer Sex Reference Guide

(For updated information, please consult the Centers for Disease Control and Prevention website at cdc.gov.)

Unprotected Anal/Vaginal Contact

High Risk	Moderate Risk	No Risk	N/A
Bacterial vaginosis	Hepatitis C	None	Lice/Scabies
Chlamydia			
Gonorrhea			
Hepatitis A			
Hepatitis B			
Herpes			
HIV			
HPV			
Syphilis			

Unprotected Penis/Vagina Sex

High Risk	Moderate Risk	No Risk	N/A
Bacterial vaginosis	Hepatitis A	None	None
Chlamydia	Hepatitis C		
Gonorrhea			
Hepatitis B			
Herpes			
HIV			
HPV			
Lice/Scabies			
Syphilis			

Unprotected Anal Sex

High Risk	Moderate Risk	No Risk	N/A
Gonorrhea	None	Bacterial vaginosis	None
Hepatitis B		Chlamydia	
Hepatitis C		Hepatitis A	
Herpes			
HIV			
HPV			
Lice/Scabies			
Syphilis			

Sharing Anything That Comes Into Insertable Genital Contact (Sex Toys, Fetish Items, Insertables)

High Risk	Moderate Risk	No Risk	N/A
Chlamydia	Bacterial vaginosis	None	None
Gonorrhea	Hepatitis A		
Hepatitis B	Hepatitis C		
Syphilis	Herpes		
	HIV		
	HPV		
	Lice/Scabies		
	Vaginitis		

Deep Kissing and Sharing External Genital Contact Items
(Rubber Panties, Items That May Pass Moisture or Fluids, Etc.)

High Risk	Moderate Risk	No Risk	N/A
None	Gonorrhea	Chlamydia	Vaginitis
	Hepatitis B	Hepatitis A	
	Herpes	Hepatitis C	
	HPV	HIV	
	Lice/Scabies		
	Syphilis		
	Bacterial vaginosis (N/A for kissing without vaginal contact)		

*Dry kissing: no risk

Ejaculation in Eyes*

High Risk	Moderate Risk	No Risk	N/A
Chlamydia	HIV	Hepatitis A	Bacterial vaginosis
Gonorrhea	HPV	Hepatitis C	Lice/Scabies
Hepatitis B			Vaginitis
Herpes			
Syphilis			

*Chlamydia, gonorrhea, and syphilis will cause conjunctivitis

Ejaculation on Exterior of Female Genitals

High Risk	Moderate Risk	No Risk	N/A
Gonorrhea	Chlamydia	None	Bacterial vaginosis
Hepatitis A	Hepatitis C		Lice/Scabies
Hepatitis B	HIV		Vaginitis
Herpes			
HPV			
Syphilis			

Ejaculation in Nose

High Risk	Moderate Risk	No Risk	N/A
Chlamydia	HIV	None	Bacterial vaginosis
Gonorrhea	HPV		Hepatitis A
Hepatitis B			Hepatitis C
Herpes			Lice/Scabies
Syphilis			Vaginitis

Anal to Oral Contact (Penis, Insertable, or Sex Toy)

High Risk	Moderate Risk	No Risk	N/A
Gonorrhea	Chlamydia	Lice/Scabies	Bacterial vaginosis
Hepatitis A	Hepatitis C		Vaginitis
Hepatitis B	HIV		
Herpes			
HPV			
Syphilis			

Unprotected Fellatio (Giving)

High Risk	Moderate Risk	No Risk	N/A
Gonorrhea	Chlamydia	Hepatitis A	Bacterial vaginosis
Hepatitis B	HIV	Hepatitis C	Vaginitis
Herpes	HPV		
Syphilis	Lice/Scabies		

Unprotected Fellatio (Receiving)

High Risk	Moderate Risk	No Risk	N/A
Gonorrhea	Chlamydia	Hepatitis A	Bacterial vaginosis
Herpes	Hepatitis B	Hepatitis C	Vaginitis
Syphilis	HIV		
	HPV		
	Lice/Scabies		

Unprotected Cunnilingus (Giving)

High Risk	Moderate Risk	No Risk	N/A
Gonorrhea	HIV	Chlamydia	Bacterial vaginosis
Herpes	HPV	Hepatitis A	Vaginitis
Syphilis	Lice/Scabies	Hepatitis B	
		Hepatitis C	

Unprotected Cunnilingus (Receiving)

High Risk	Moderate Risk	No Risk	N/A
Gonorrhea	Chlamydia	Hepatitis A	Bacterial vaginosis
Herpes	HPV	Hepatitis B	Vaginitis
Syphilis	Lice/Scabies	Hepatitis C	
		HIV	

Unprotected Rimming (Giving)

High Risk	Moderate Risk	No Risk	N/A
Gonorrhea	Chlamydia	None	Bacterial vaginosis
Hepatitis A	Hepatitis C		Vaginitis
Hepatitis B	HIV		
Herpes	Lice/Scabies		
HPV			
Syphilis			

Unprotected Rimming (Receiving)

High Risk	Moderate Risk	No Risk	N/A
Gonorrhea	Chlamydia	Hepatitis A	Bacterial vaginosis
Hepatitis B	Hepatitis C		Vaginitis
Herpes	HIV		
Syphilis	HPV		
	Lice/Scabies		

Fetish Sex Rule #3: Play Safe With Your Ass

When we crave the wonderfully intense feeling of anal stimulation, we often don't have exactly the toy we wished we had handy. No doubt you've heard urban legends about people going to the ER with all manner of odd and potentially lethal items lodged in their rectums—and unfortunately, quite a few of these stories are true. Don't make a hasty decision; make sure you only stick things in your butt that are safe, easy to retrieve, and made for anal play. Toys made for anal play will have a flared base, much wider around than the rest of the toy. Make the right choice when you stimulate your ass. Even if you're ashamed or unwilling to admit what you like, we're talking about avoiding embarrassment and serious injury.

Always use lots of lubrication—the skin around the anus tears easily, but won't if it's lubed enough. Never put something in your butt—or anywhere near your butt—that has sharp edges, can possibly break, shatter or crack, or doesn't have a significantly flared base for easy retrieval. A tiny cut inside your rectum can easily become infected with fecal matter and can lead to more serious infections involving other organs in your body and could lead to life-threatening situations if left untreated.

The ring of anal muscles likes to grab and pull inside anything you put in, and these muscles are involuntary, meaning you have no control over them. A lubed anal sphincter will pull in anything you put inside, and if you can't grab it safely to pull it back out, you're off to becoming another urban legend. Shampoo bottles and Barbie dolls are right out—get the right toy, such as a butt plug or dildo that's made for anal use. Sometimes if you "lose" an item, you can bear down and push it out, but if it's past a certain point in your lower colon you'll need professional (medical) help to get it back out. If you lose an item and you can't get it out after a few tries, get help at the hospital immediately—don't even try to get it out yourself if it breaks, has a motor, or has sharp edges.

Fetish Sex Rule #4: Know Your Bondage and BDSM Basics

- Always have a "safeword." A safeword is a word that you and your partner both agree means "stop now." Pick an unusual word you seldom use, and avoid using "no" or "stop" in case you'd like to feign resistance to your predicament. Everyone should have a safeword, and some people have a word for "stop" and a separate word for "a little less, thank you." Stoplight colors—red, yellow, and green—are very popular. If one of you uses the safeword, stop the scene and switch activities to cuddling, snacking, and talking.
- Learn how to tie a knot and how to untie it as well. Read *The Erotic Bondage Handbook* by Jay Wiseman if you're going to engage in any kind of bondage or restriction play. Read Hardy Haberman's *Family Jewels* to learn the safe and fun points of male genital bondage and torture.
- Keep medical scissors handy in case your knots are too tight, your bondage is painful or cuts off circulation, or your lover needs to get out of whatever it is, fast.
- Don't lay anyone on bound or cuffed wrists. Tie a long brightly colored ribbon to your handcuff key so it's impossible to lose, and never tie anything around the throat, ever. If you gag your sweetie, establish a physical safeword, and watch for jaw cramp or too much in the mouth, which might cause a gag reflex. And remember—if you restrain

someone in public, you'll probably wind up in jail.

- If punishment fits your scene, and intense sensations like clamps, spanking, whipping, paddling and other types of pain are what you want, it is absolutely required that you carefully discuss what is going to happen. It must be absolutely clear that you both want to try it, and the receiving partner must give explicit consent.
- Start, and always, go slow.
- Never try to have sex (even solo masturbation) in a BDSM club or fetish event unless it's absolutely clear that this is okay.
- Never ask a dominatrix for sex. To learn more about finding a dominatrix, read *The Ultimate Guide to Sexual Fantasy* by (me!) Violet Blue.

Fetish Sex Rule #5: Love Your Gift

Having a sexual fetish is a very refined, fun, special, and exciting way to enjoy sex. Never treat yourself badly because of your fetish (unless it turns you on), and don't be ashamed of who you are, fetishes and all. Don't let people who don't understand make you feel bad. Never forget that you're not alone. Don't feel lonely because you understand yourself better than anyone else; you're way ahead of the rest of the world by being sexually self-reliant, and you know how to share what makes you hot with other people only when you're ready (and when they're deserving). Relish your fetish, love it, roll with it and even if you feel lonely make yourself feel good once in a while with a hot fetish masturbation session. Your fetish is a gift: many people spend most of their lives looking for the things that turn them on, and never find it. Love your gift.

Panty Tease
Thomas Roche

They'd been playing with tease-and-denial—it had been going on for two weeks now. Fourteen days since they started, eleven since his last orgasm.

Erin was usually an immediate-gratification kind of girl, so she never would have gone this far if he hadn't long ago confessed that being teased into a frenzy—and denied any form of sexual release—was his biggest, fondest fantasy, one that drove him crazy, one that never failed—ironically enough—to bring him quickly to orgasm when he was fantasizing.

But that was out of the question, now—this was the fourteenth day of their scene, and he had obeyed her directive: No masturbation. Not even a stroke. No masturbation, Carl, and you're not going to fuck me.

Every night when they saw each other, she teased him. It had started with the sexy lingerie, short skirts, high heels, Erin flashing him a little as he made dinner, coming up behind him and easing her hand down his pants to caress his ass and, sometimes, stroke his cock. It had progressed as days passed without his orgasm, his cock hard and aching as she paraded through the kitchen in her skimpies, even played with herself on the counter while he diced zucchini and sliced carrots. Then dinner, with her half-clad at the table and him feeling the stroke of her bare foot in his crotch in between bites.

After dinner, there were the lap dances—her writhing for him, grinding against him, brushing her breasts in his face, allowing him to suckle her tits, caress her ass, even slide his finger into her G-string to feel how wet she was. Sometimes she would prop herself up on the coffee table, legs spread, and stroke herself until she came—always reminding him to sit on his hands unless he was touching her. He could not touch himself. Then, when she was satisfied, she would strip off her lingerie and they would go to bed, where he would be allowed to service her for hours with his tongue, until she'd had all she could take. They would cuddle up naked together and she would doze off, and Carl would be left hungry and throbbing, aching to fuck her, aching to jerk off.

But he didn't—he would fall asleep, finally, hurting with his need, wanting it, wanting more, wanting to be denied.

After three days he was so aroused that he actually had a wet dream—his first since puberty. She awakened to a spurt of come on her belly. She laughed and punished him by making him sleep on the couch, and wouldn't allow him to touch her for three days. The teasing continued, from a distance, her always satisfying herself. Then, finally, she allowed him to service her again, and he swore he would never come again without permission.

And he hadn't, not even now, when for the last three days she had denied him even the pleasure of servicing him—and, in a storm of wicked inspiration, she had him washing her panties.

They were delicate garments, these, all satin and lace, skimpy and fragrant. Fourteen of them, the sexiest thongs and French-cut panties she owned, and he had been teased with each and every one of them. He could vividly remember how she'd looked—dancing in front of him, or spread on the coffee table, or stretched out on the bed waiting for him to delicately slide her panties over her hips, down her thighs, over her ankles. He remembered each scene, recognized each pair of panties. Each held a charge that made his cock harder than ever.

As he prepared to hand wash the panties in the basin in the garage sink, he couldn't resist. He took the skimpiest one, the tiny white lace thong she'd worn when she'd teased him the first time—and he brought it to his face. He drew deeply of her scent. Two weeks on, the scent was ripe, musky, filthy in more ways than one. The heady aroma sent a pulse through his body, and he gave a tiny but audible moan, glancing over his shoulder as if to make sure she wasn't watching. She hadn't ordered him not to sniff her panties—but she hadn't said he could.

Erin's cunt smelled like sex—raw, unadulterated sex, and he couldn't resist the fragrance. He slipped the crotch into his mouth and suckled on it, tasting her. He longed to slip his tongue inside her. Three long days it had been since he tasted her cunt fresh—and this taste, aged and sharp, made him swoon.

He slipped the white thong, now moist with his spittle, out of his mouth and immersed it in the basin. Rather than scrubbing it, though, he moved on to the next garment—a skimpy black lace G-string she'd worn when she'd spread herself on the coffee table for the first time, and pleasured herself as she made him watch. He moaned as he sniffed it—she'd been very turned on that night, very wet, and the scent still lingered, more powerful than on the white thong. He breathed deeply, her aroma like a drug, and bit into the crotch of them desperately. He could taste her. Stronger than before. Stronger, it seemed, than he tasted her when he buried his tongue in her sex. He moaned. He reached for his cock, getting the top button of his jeans undone, stopping himself only at the last moment. He took another deep breath and, whimpering, slid the black panties under the water.

He felt faint when he picked up the next pair. Red—slut red, stripper red, tease red—and thin, without a cotton crotch, her smell suffusing the thin satin and the thinner lace. His dizziness mounted. God, he fucking wanted her. He had to touch himself. He had to touch his cock. He just *had* to touch his fucking cock.

But he didn't—he held himself back. He tasted her, suckling and nursing on the pussy-infused satin fabric, tears forming in his eyes as he resisted the urge to masturbate. He slid the spittle-moist garment under the soapy water and turned his attention to the next pair of panties.

The crotchless ones. Crotchless so she could prop herself on the coffee table and spread herself to show him how wet she was. Crotchless so she could fuck herself with a dildo while she made him sit on his hands, and squirm, and whimper like a dog. Crotchless, so she could rub herself and laugh when she saw him shuddering all over, aching to come— aching to fuck her.

He inhaled and almost passed out from the delectable fragrance. Every cell of his body hummed with its power. He huffed her panties like a kid huffing glue—it was a savage feeling, coursing through his body, overwhelming need turning swiftly to unbearable agony. He needed her. He wanted her. She was everything—God, how he wanted to fuck her.

"My, my," he heard Erin's voice from behind him. "You *are* in a bad way. Reduced to sniffing panties." He turned to regard her; he had been so absorbed in her underwear that he hadn't noticed her entering the garage, seating herself on the stool behind him.

She was wearing a simple wrap skirt, clasped in the front. When she spread her legs and opened it, he saw that she wasn't wearing a stitch underneath.

He didn't need to be told. He was down on his knees in an instant, his mouth pressed to her sex, his tongue finding her cleft and settling on her swollen clit, servicing her. The taste was sharp. She was very aroused.

"Touch your dick," she told him breathlessly as he licked her. "But don't jerk off."

He obeyed, taking out his cock and holding it, squeezing gently, but not stroking. Oh God, just a few strokes would bring him off, but he didn't allow himself that. The heightened agony only made him lick her more fervently.

She came within minutes, moaning and writhing on his tongue, biting her finger as she looked down at him. When she was finished, she gently pushed him away and said, "Take your hand off your cock."

He twisted up inside, ambivalent. Half of him had hoped she would finally relent and allow him to stroke himself to orgasm. The other half of him thrilled when she ordered him not to.

He obediently put his cock away as Erin got off the stool, closed her wrap skirt, and headed for the garage door.

"Be sure to scrub," she said over her shoulder as she left. "They're filthy. But then, you already knew that." Her voice was musical.

Shaking all over, humming with unsatisfied arousal, he returned to the basin. He selected the next pair of panties from the pile...and brought it to his face, inhaling her scent.

Chapter 11
Resources

Chapter 1: Guess My Fetish
Books
Best Fetish Erotica, edited by Cara Bruce
Deviant Desires: Incredibly Strange Sex by Katharine Gates
Fakir Musafar: Spirit + Flesh by Fakir Musafar
Re/Search #12: Modern Primitives by V. Vale
Sweet Life: Erotic Fantasies for Couples 1 and 2 and *Taboo*
    by Violet Blue
Wild Side Sex: The Book of Kink by Midori

Websites
craigslist.org (for meeting and networking with others,
    also events)
deviantdesires.com
en.wikipedia.org/wiki/Sexual_fetishism

Fetbot, "fetish resource guide" (mostly commercial):
fetbot.com
Fleshbot: fleshbot.com (search by fetish topic for an array
of sites and reviews)
Index of fetish galleries:
http://directory.google.com/Top/Adult/Image_
Galleries/
sexuality.org/l/fetish/
tribe.net (lots of communities and discussions)

Thousands of individual fetish websites can be found at
http://dir.yahoo.com/Business_and_Economy/
Shopping_and_Services/Sex/Adult_Galleries/.
Fewer sites, though less commerce-oriented than the
index above, are at http://dir.yahoo.com/Society_
and_Culture/Sexuality/Fetishes_and_Fantasies/.
Personal pages on this index:
http://dir.yahoo.com/Society_and_Culture/
Sexuality/Activities_and_Practices/

Chapter 2: Sexual Secrets
Books
The Erotic Mind by Jack Morin
For Yourself: The Fulfillment of Female Sexuality by Lonnie
Barbach, Ph. D.
*Sex Talk: Uncensored Exercises for Exploring What Really
Turns You On* by Lauren Dockett and Aline P.
Zoldbrod
*The Survivor's Guide to Sex: How to Have an Empowering Sex
Life After Child Sexual Abuse* by Staci Haines (also see
Staci's video: *Healing Sex: Finding Pleasure and Intimacy
After Surviving Sexual Abuse*)

The Ultimate Guide to Sexual Fantasy by Violet Blue

Website for more healing information: generationfive.org

Chapter 3: Fetishes and Sex
Books
Come Hither: A Common Sense Guide to Kinky Sex by
    Gloria Brame
*For Each Other: Sharing Sexual Intimacy and Turn-Ons:
    Pleasing Yourself While You Please Your Lover* by
    Lonnie Barbach, Ph. D.
Sensuous Magic: A Guide to S/M for Adventurous Couples
    by Patrick Califia

Chapter 4: The Heart of Fetish: Role-Play
Books
Exhibitionism for the Shy: Show Off, Dress Up, and Talk Hot
    by Carol Queen
*The Fine Art of Erotic Talk: How to Entice, Excite and
    Enchant Your Lover With Words* by Bonnie Gabriel

Shopping Websites
costumes.org
ebay.com
sexycostumestore.com

Also: Used Panty Portal, usedpantyportal.com

Chapter 5: Fetish Dressing
Corsets and Tight-Lacing
Books
The Corset: A Cultural History by Valerie Steele
Fetish Fashion: Undressing the Corset by Larry Utley and
Autumn Carey-Adamme

Websites
The Corset Site: corset.dk/
The Corset College: corsetcollege.co.funpic.de/
European Corset Society: eucosy.org/
Long Island Staylace Association: staylace.com/

Less common fetishwear items:
JT's Stockroom: stockroom.com

Female Latex-Mask Fetish, aka Masking
Closet Monster: closetmonster.net
Kerry's links: maskon.com/kerry/links.htm
Maskon: maskon.com
Rubbersisters: rubbersisters.de/

Cosplay
American Cosplay Paradise: acparadise.com
Cosplay: cosplay.com
Cosplay Lab: cosplaylab.com
Cute Cosplay Angels: sexyangels.blogspot.com

Going Out: Parties and Events
Eros Guide: eros-guide.com/events.htm
Jane's Guide: janesguide.com
        (site uses frames; look under Jane's Regional Guide:
•your state or country•/Night Clubs/Resorts)

San Francisco
DomDominion: domdominion.com
Exotic Erotic: exoticeroticball.com
Folsom Street Fair/Up Your Alley (Dore Alley) Fair:
    folsomstreetfair.com
Slick Fetish Ball: clubslick.com

New York
Black and Blue Ball: blackandblueball.com

Germany
German Fetish Ball: german-fetish-ball.com

UK
Skin Two Rubber Ball: skintworubberball.com

Leather
Books
Leather and Latex Care by Kelly Thibault
Leatherfolk, edited by Mark Thompson
*Leathersex: A Guide for the Curious Outsider and the Serious
    Player* by Joseph W. Bean
Leathersex Q&A by Joseph W. Bean
*Ties That Bind: The SM/Leather/Fetish Erotic Style: Issues,
    Commentaries and Advice* by Guy Baldwin and Joseph
    W. Bean

Websites
The Leather Journal: theleatherjournal.com/index.html

Rubber

Books

Making Latex Clothes by Sian-Kate Mooney
Leather and Latex Care by Kelly Thibault
Rubber: Fun, Fashion, Fetish by Janet Bloor and John D.
   Sinclair

Magazines (Print)

Blue Blood
Demonia
Fetish Realm
Heavy Rubber
Marquis
Secret
Skin Two
Ritual
Taboo

Websites

3xl: Lust, Love & Latex: lustlovelatex.com
Blue Blood: blueblood.net
Fetish Realm Magazine: fetish-realm.com
The International Association of Rubberists: rubberist.net/
Marquis Magazine (German): marquis.de
The Rubber Fetish Site (M4M, great images of men):
   fetishball.com/
Secret Magazine: secretmag.com
Skin Two Magazine: skintwo.com

Rubber and fetish fashion community network: Check out
the wide variety of fetish links in the "rubberdex" at
rubberist.net

Chapter 6: Human Animals
Pony Play
Books

The United States Pony Club Manual of Horsemanship : Basics for Beginners/D Level, edited by Susan E. Harris and Ruth Ring Harvie

Websites

Academy Incorporated:
www.tawse.com/html/homeframe.html
Equus Eroticus: equuseroticus.com
The Human Equine: thehumanequine.com
Lord Saber's Pony Play FAQ:
tdl.com/~thawley/ponyfaq.htm
Riding Women (male ponies): ridingwomen.com/home.html
The Stampede: the-stampede.com

Dogs and Pups
Books

Woof! Perspectives Into the Erotic Care and Training of the Human Dog by Michael Daniels

Websites

International Puppy & Trainer Contest:
intlpuppycontest.org
Leatherdog (M4M): leatherdog.com (extensive links, including community resources for many types of animal play)

Shopping sites for a variety of human animals:
JT's Stockroom: stockroom.com
Mr. S Leathers: mr-s-leather-fetters.com

Other Animals and Fantasy Creatures
BDSM Animal Training (dog, pony, pig):
 mybdsm.com/pages/animal/intro.html
Pet Girls (cute paysite): petgirls.com
The Water Hole (ponies and dogs): water-hole.com/

Plushies and Furries
Books
The American Journal of Anthropomorphics by Darrell
 Benvenuto

Websites
Anthrocon (convention): anthrocon.org
FurNation: furnation.com
Furry Grand Central: furcen.org/fgc/
Mascot Costumes: mascotscostumes.com/
Tigerden: tigerden.com

Also: Search "mascot costumes" on Amazon.com and eBay

Chapter 7: Cross-Dressing and Sissies
Books
Dominance by Mistress Loreli
The Lazy Crossdresser by Charles Anders
Miss Vera's Cross Dress for Success and *Miss Vera's Finishing
 School for Boys Who Want to be Girls* by Veronica Vera
My Husband Betty: Love, Sex, and Life with a Crossdresser by
 Helen Boyd
Out & About: The Emancipated Crossdresser and *7 Secrets of
 Successful Crossdressers* by Lacey Leigh

Gender (Mostly Male-to-Female) Exploration
Books
Best Transgender Erotica, edited by Hanne Blank and
    Raven Kaldera
The Gender Frontier by Mariette Pathy Allen
*My Gender Workbook: How to Become a Real Man, a Real
    Woman, the Real You, or Something Else Entirely* by Kate
    Bornstein
The Tranny Guide by Vicki Lee

Shopping and Resources
All Heels for Men: allheelsformen.com
The Breast Form Store: thebreastformstore.com
Classic Curves International: clcrv.com
Cross-Dress Boutique: cross-dress.com
Crossdressers International: cdinyc.org
The Fantasy Girl: thefantasygirl.com
Frishman's Intimate Apparel: frish.com
Miss Vera's Finishing School: missvera.com
Queen Fashions: queenfashions.com
Tranny Fest: Transgender/Transgenre Cinema:
    trannyfest.com
Tranny International: trannyinternational.com
Transgender Forum: tgforum.com
Versatile Fashions: versatile-fashions.com
WayOut Publishing: wayout-publishing.com

Sissies and Sissy Maids
Books
A Charm School for Sissy Maids by Mistress Lorelei
The Compleat Spanker by Lady Green

Websites
Club Sissy: clubsissy.com
Fetish Flame podcast interview (audio) with forced
    feminization pro, Natasha Strange:
    odeo.com/audio/64637/view
The House of Sissify: sissify.com
Humiliatrix: humiliatrix.com
Lacy's Frilly Fashions: laceys.ca
Petticoated: petticoated.com
Sissy School: sissyschool.com
Sissy Search: sissysearch.com

Chapter 8: Medical Play and Adult Babies
General Medical-Play Resources
Books
Family Jewels: A Guide to Male Genital Play and Torment
    by Hardy Haberman
Hand in the Bush: The Fine Art of Vaginal Fisting by
    Deborah Addington
Intimate Invasions: The Erotic Ins & Outs Of Enema Play
    by M.R. Strict
Juice: Electricity for Pleasure and Pain by Uncle Abdul
Sex Disasters and How to Survive Them by Charles Moser,
    PH.D., M.D., and Janet W. Hardy
The Toybag Guides, Greenery Press
*Trust, the Hand Book: A Guide to the Sensual and Spiritual
    Art of Handballing* by Bert Herrman

Medical Outfits and Uniforms
AllHeart: allheart.com
Anthony's Uniforms: anthonys-uniforms.com
Siren's Secrets: sirenssecrets.com/naughtynurses.html
Three Wishes Lingerie: threewisheslingerie.com/nurse.asp

Medical Instruments
JT's Stockroom: stockroom.com
Medical Toys (also offers uniforms and rubber):
medicaltoys.com

Play-Piercing Information
Notes on Play Piercing: sexuality.org/l/bdsm/needle.html

Adult Baby (AB) and Diaper Lovers
Diaper Incontinence Resource shop: idiaper.com
Diaper Pail Friends (shopping mommy manuals, chat,
connect, extensive links): dpf.com
Forever A Kid: foreverakid.com

Adult Thumbsucking
Thumbsucking Adults: thumbsuckingadults.com

Chapter 9: About the Body
Nice fetish link collection at Gloria Brame's site:
gloria-brame.com/kinkylinks/fetishpage2.html

Boobs
Big Boobs Sites
Big Boobs: bigboobs.bz
Breast Expansion Archive: bearchive.com
Breastlove's Babes: breastlove.blogspot.com
My Boob Site: myboobsite.com
The Overflowing Bra: overflowingbra.com
Time 4 Boobs: time4boobs.com
Tits-Out: tits-out.com

Little Boobs Site
Itty Bitty Titty Committee: tinytitty.tribe.net

Butts
Apple Bottom Girls: applebottomgirls.blogspot.com
    Hot Ass Pages: hotass.jp
Asses: sexyingapics.blogspot.com
Big Butt Magazine: bigbuttmag.com
Bounce That Ass Blog: bounce-that-ass.skyblog.com
Buttman Magazine and porn videos/sites: buttman.com

Foot and Leg Fetish
Books
All books by Elmer Batters (Amazon.com)
All books by photographer Roy Stuart (Amazon.com)

Websites
Foot Fetish Planet: foot-fetish-planet.com
Hard-Core Foot Sex: Porno-Feet.com
Leg Fetish Gallery: ffbikyaku.jp
Leg Show Magazine: legshow.com
Pantyhose Mama: pantyhosemama.com
Roy Stuart's website: roystuart.com
Serafina's Socks: serafinasox.com
Stockings HQ: stockingshq.com
Toe and Arch: toeandarch.com

Ear Fetish
Japanese Ear Fetish:
    homepage3.nifty.com/earfetish/index-top.html

Nose Fetish, or Pinocchia
Big Nose Appreciation Page: pinocchia.com/bnguy/

Big Nose FAQ: cyberium.net/bnguy/bnfaq.htm
Jim's Nose Morph Page: ohnoitsjim.iwarp.com
Pinocchia: forums.pinocchia.com

Bald Beauties, Shaved Heads, and Long Hair
Digital Hair Extensions: digital-hair-extension.com
Female Head-Shaving Blog: femaleheadshaving.web-log.nl
The Long Hair Site: tlhs.org/faq.html

Fingernails, Long-Nail Fetish
The Alarmingly Long and Dangerous Nails Page:
    members.aol.com/DC0007
Fingernail Fetish: fingernailfetish.com

Inflation
BodyInflation: bodyinflation.org
Expandemonium: expandemonium.net
The Inflatable Clothing/Body Inflation Website:
    icb2e.expandemonium.net/body.aspx

Scars
Film: *Crash,* directed by David Cronenberg

Pregnancy and Lactation
Books
Breastfeeding and Human Lactation by Jan Riordan

Websites
Bambi's Zone: stormrszone.com
Bellius Maximus: belliusmaximus.com
Naked Preganant: naked-pregnant.com
PG-13: ninpuchan.dreamhost.com

Fat Fetish
BBW Network: bbwnetwork.com
Big Cuties: bigcuties.com
Bodacious Magazine: bodaciousmagazine.com
Cute Plumper: cuteplumper.com
Large and Lovely: largeandlovely.com
Southern Charms: southern-charms.com
We Love Big Girls: welovebiggirls.blogspot.com

Chastity Belts
Chastity UK: chastity-uk.co.uk

Wet and Messy Play
Messy Online: messy-online.com
WAM Productions: wamproduction.com
Splosh!: splosh.co.uk

Smoking
Andrew Blake videos: andrewblake.com
IRL Exposed: irlexposed.net
Smoking Fetish Links: links.smokesigs.com

Amputees and Devotees
ABC Links: abc-links.com/index.php
Ampulove free pics:
    ampulove.com/freepictures/freepictures.htm
Cutoff Gallery: cutoff.slyp.net
Devguide: devguide.org
Sex Toy Body Parts: adameve.com, look for "Vivid Video"
    toys

Bodily Fluids
Fully Clothed Pissing: fullyclothedpissing.com

Public Pissgirl: public-pissgirl.com
Shitgirl inPublic: shitgirl-in-public.com
Sneeze Fetish Videos: www.5a.biglobe.ne.jp/~kago-
    usu/KushamiRoom/kushami-E.html
Snot Girls: snotgirls.com
Vomit Online: vomitonline.com
Wet Set Magazine: wetset.net

Forniphilia
House of Gord, the "home of ultra-bondage" is a shrine
for extreme rubber fetishists and forniphiliacs (human
rubberized furniture): houseofgord.com

Giantesses, Trampling, and Being Crushed
Giantess Zone: giantesszone.com
GTS Feet and Crush: feet-crush.com
Maxcat's Giantess Realm: maxcatsrealm.com

Balloons and Looners
Balloon Girls: balloongirls.com
Loonerz: loonerz.com

Human Mannequins and Robots
Fleshbot Resource Listing: fleshbot.com/sex/video/
    asfr-robot-fetish-video-112305.php
Fucking Machines: fuckingmachines.com
The Living Mannequin Circle: freezemodeling.com
Sybian: sybian.com

Midgets
Sexy Midgets: sexy-midgets.com

Tickling
Books
Erotic Tickling by Michael Moran

Videos
Converted to Ticking by Maria Beatty, bleuproductions.com

Websites
Tickling Cartoon Fetish Gallery:
	angel.ne.jp/~defiant/tickling_gallery.html
Tickling Media Forum: ticklingforum.com

Sleeping
Somnophilia: Sex With Sleeping Girls: somnophilia.com

Carrying or "Lift and Carry"
Sleeping Beauties: sleeping-beauties.com

Necrophilia
Necrobabes link list: necrobabes.org
Vicki's Necrobabe pages: necrobabes.org/vicki/home.htm

Chapter 10: Fetish Sex Essentials

General Fetish Sex Resources
Books
Consensual Sadomasochism, Second Edition by Bill Henkin
	and Sybil Holiday
The Guide to Getting It On! by Paul Joannides
*The Erotic Bondage Handbook and S/M 101: A Realistic
	Introduction* by Jay Wiseman

The Seductive Art of Japanese Bondage by Midori and Craig
   Morey
*SlaveCraft: Roadmaps for Erotic Servitude: Principles, Skills,
   and Tools* by a Grateful Slave with Guy Baldwin, M.S.

Safer Sex
Centers for Disease Control National AIDS Clearinghouse
P.O. Box 6003, Rockville, MD 20849; (800) 342-AIDS;
cdcnac.com

Cetra Latex-Free Supplies
A product site for latex-free gear, catering mainly to the
medical community (because so many medical profession-
als end up with latex allergies). Sells to individuals. Nice
site-wide search.
(888) LATEX-NO; (510) 848-3345; latexfree.com

Condomania
Exhaustive site that sells virtually every condom under
the sun, with fun facts, lots of condom information, and a
helpful condom shopping guide.
(800) 9CONDOM; (800) 926-6366; condomania.com

National AIDS Hotline
(800) 342-2437

National STD Hotline
(800) 227-8922

Safer Sex Page
safersex.org

San Francisco Sex Information
Sex information and referral switchboard that provides free, nonjudgmental, anonymous, accurate information about anything sex related. Hours: 3 P.M.–9 P.M., PT, Mon.–Fri. They also answer email questions.
(877)-472 7374; (415) 989-SFSI; sfsi.org

About the Author

Violet Blue is an author, editor, robot mechanic, female porn expert, and professional pro-porn pundit. She is girl Friday contributor at Fleshbot.com, an author at Metblogs SF and a correspondent at Geek Entertainment TV by day, and a human blog by night. Violet has been a published sex columnist and trained professional sex educator since 1998, a member of Survival Research Laboratories since 1996, and she frequently lectures to students about human sexuality in UC's and community teaching institutions. She is the editor of six erotic anthologies and the author of five sex education books, two of which have been best-selling sex-advice books since their release and have been translated into French, Spanish, and Russian. Her influences are J.G. Ballard, David Sedaris, John Waters, Emir Kusturica, Mark Pauline, A.M. Homes, Patrick Califia, and Patty Hearst. She has been interviewed, featured, and quoted as an expert by more magazine, web, television, and radio outlets than can be listed here, including *The Wall Street Journal*, *Newsweek*, NPR, CNN, *Wired*, *Esquire*, and Web MD. For more information visit her website tinynibbles.com or listen to her podcast, Open Source Sex.

About Thomas Roche

Thomas Roche's erotic stories have appeared in hundreds of magazines, websites, and books, including the Best American Erotica series, the Best New Erotica series, and many other anthologies. His books include three volumes of the Noirotica series and the short story collections *Dark Matter* and, with Alison Tyler, *His and Hers*. He is currently Managing Editor of Eros Zine (eros-zine.com). He can also be found online at skidroche.com and livejournal.com/users/thomasroche.

Also available from
Daedalus Publishing Company

Wild Side Sex- The Book of Kink
Educational, Sensual, and Entertaining Essays
Tired of standing on the sexual sidelines? Wonder what it's like to be a real "kink" adventurer? Let the world famous Midori take you by the hand (or by the collar if that's your pleasure) and lead you into the thick of it. This delightfully twisted guide takes erotic adventure to a personal level and exposes some of Midori's most helpful, empowering secrets. **$18.00**

Debbie's Gift
An Erotic Story of Female Dominance
After a night of lovemaking, lawyer husband Ron agrees to become wife Debbie's slave. The next morning, a harsh reality sets in as Ron is "netted" and carted away to be trained in the arts of sexual slavery at a high tech facility. A tale of sacrifice, and, ultimately, love, Debbie's Gift is a dark, thrilling free fall of a sci-fi/erotic ride. By Amity Harris. Fiction. **$18.00**

Nominated for the 2004 Stonewall Book Award!!!
Painfully Obvious
An Irreverent & Unauthorized Manual for Leather/SM
Robert Davolt's new anthology takes an unorthodox look at leather relationships, community, contests, business, tradition, history and leadership. Inside perspective and practical tips on "What To Wear," "Leather On The Cheap" and "Passing The Bar," are delivered with authoritative research and barbed humor. **$16.95**

10th Anniversary Edition, Lambda Literary-Award Nominated
Leatherfolk
Radical Sex, People, Politics, and Practice
Edited by Mark Thompson, this anthology has become a classic, must read book on human sexuality and identity. The diverse, contributors look at the history of the gay and lesbian underground, how radical sex practice relates to their spirituality, and what S/M means to them personally. **$17.00**

Spirit + Flesh
Fakir Musafar's Photo Book
After 50 years photographing Fakir Musafar's own body and the play of others, here is a deluxe retrospective collection of amazing images you'll find nowhere else... 296 oversize pages, three pounds worth! This book is a "must have" for all serious body modifiers, tattoo and piercing studios. **$49.50**

Urban Aboriginals
A Celebration of Leathersexuality – 20th Anniversary Edition
As relevant today as when it was written 20 years ago, author Geoff Mains takes an intimate view of the gay male leather community. Explore the spiritual, sexual, emotional, cultural and physiological aspects that make this "scene" one of the most prominent yet misunderstood subcultures in our society. **$15.95**

Carried Away
An S/M Romance
In david stein's first novel, steamy Leathersex is only the beginning when a cocky, jaded bottom and a once-burned Master come together for some no-strings bondage and S/M. Once the scene is over, a deeper hunger unexpectedly awakens, and they begin playing for much higher stakes. **$19.95**

Ties That Bind
The SM/Leather/Fetish Erotic Style- Issues, Commentaries and Advice
The early writings of well-known psychotherapist and respected member of the leather community Guy Baldwin have been compiled to create this SM classic. Second edition. **$16.95**

SlaveCraft
Roadmaps for Erotic Servitude Principles, Skills and Tools
Guy Baldwin, author of *Ties That Bind*, joins forces with a grateful slave to produce this gripping and personal account on the subject of consensual slavery. **$15.95**

My Private Life
Real Experiences of a Dominant Woman
Within these pages, the author, Mistress Nan, allows the reader a brief glimpse into the true private life of an erotically dominant woman. Each scene is vividly detailed and reads like the finest erotica, but knowing that these scenes really occurred as written adds to the sexual excitement they elicit. Second edition. **$16.95**

The Master's Manual
A Handbook of Erotic Dominance
In this book, author Jack Rinella examines various aspects of erotic dominance, including S/M, safety, sex, erotic power, techniques and more. The author speaks in a clear, frank, and nonjudgmental way to anyone with an interest in the erotic Dominant/submissive dynamic. **$15.95**

The Compleat Slave
Creating and Living and Erotic Dominant/submissive Lifestyle
In this highly anticipated follow up to The Master's Manual, author Jack Rinella continues his in-depth exploration of Dominant/submissive relationships. **$15.95**

Consensual Sadomasochism
How to Talk About It and How to Do It Safely
Authors William A. Henkin, Ph. D. and Sybil Holiday, CCHT combine their extensive professional credentials with deep personal experience in this unique examination of erotic consensual sadomasochism. Second edition. **$17.95**

Chainmale: 3SM
A Unique View of Leather Culture
Author Don Bastian brings his experiences to print with this fast paced account of one man's experience with his own sexuality and eventual involvement in a loving and successful three-way kink relationship. **$13.95**

Leathersex
A Guide for the Curious Outsider and the Serious Player
Written by renowned S/M author Joseph Bean, this book gives guidance to one popular style of erotic play which the author calls 'leathersex'- sexuality that may include S/M, bondage, role playing, sensual physical stimulation and fetish, to name just a few. Second edition. **$16.95**

Leathersex Q&A
Questions About Leathersex and the Leather Lifestyle Answered
In this interesting and informative book, author Joseph Bean answers a wide variety of questions about leathersex sexuality. Each response is written with the sensitivity and insight only someone with a vast amount of experience in this style of sexuality could provide. **$16.95**

Beneath The Skins
The New Spirit and Politics of the Kink Community
This book by Ivo Dominguez, Jr. examines the many issues facing the modern leather/SM/fetish community. This special community is coming of age, and this book helps to pave the way for all who are a part of it. Second Edition. **$14.00**

Leather and Latex Care
How to Keep Your Leather and Latex Looking Great
This concise book by Kelly J. Thibault gives the reader all they need to know to keep their leather and latex items in top shape. While clothing is the focus of this book, tips are also given to those using leather and latex items in their erotic play. This book is a must for anyone investing in leather or latex. Second Edition. **$11.00**

Between The Cracks
The Daedalus Anthology of Kinky Verse
Editor Gavin Dillard has collected the most exotic of the erotic of the poetic pantheon, from the fetishes of Edna St. Vincent Millay to the howling of Ginsberg, lest any further clues be lost *between the cracks*. **$18.95**

The Leather Contest Guide
A Handbook for Promoters, Contestants, Judges and Titleholders
International Mr. Leather and Mr. National Leather Association contest winner Guy Baldwin is the author of this truly complete guide to the leather contest. Second edition. **$14.95**

Ordering Information

Phone
213.484.3882

Email
info@daedaluspublishing.com

Mail
Daedalus Publishing Company, 2807 Sunset Blvd., Los Angeles, CA 90026

Payment
All major credit cards are accepted. Via *email or regular mail*, indicate type of card, card number, expiration date, name of cardholder as shown on card, and billing address of the cardholder. Also include the mailing address where you wish your order to be sent. Orders via regular mail may include payment by money order or check, but may be held until the check clears. Make checks or money orders payable to "Daedalus Publishing Company." *Do not send cash.*

Tax and shipping
California residents, add 8.25% sales tax to the total price of the books you are ordering. *All* orders should include a $4.25 shipping charge for the first book, plus $1.00 for each additional book added to the total of the order.

Over 21 Statement
Since many of our publications deal with sexuality issues, please include a signed statement that you are at least 21 years of age with any order. Also include such a statement with any email order.